THE
HEALTHY
WOMAN
1994

THE
HEALTHY
WOMAN
1994

from **PREVENTION** Magazine Health Books and
the Rodale Center for Women's Health

edited by Alice Feinstein

Rodale Press, Emmaus, Pennsylvania

This book is being published simultaneously by Rodale Press as *The Healthy Woman*.

Copyright © 1994 by Rodale Press, Inc.

Illustrations copyright © 1994 by Linda Bleck

Printed in the United States of America on acid-free ∞, recycled paper ♻

ISBN 0–87596–196–7 hardcover
ISSN 1070–4361

4 6 8 10 9 7 5 3   hardcover

—————— OUR MISSION ——————

We publish books that empower people's lives.

—————— RODALE 🌿 BOOKS ——————

THE HEALTHY WOMAN 1994

Editor: Alice Feinstein
Research Chief: Ann Gossy Yermish
Permissions Coordinator: Anita Small
Researcher: Deborah Pedron
Cover Designer: Debra Sfetsios
Cover Photographer: Chris Harvey/Tony Stone Images
Book Designer: Karen C. Heard
Illustrator: Linda Bleck
Copy Editor: Jane Sherman
Office Staff: Roberta Mulliner, Mary Lou Stephen, Julie Kehs

CONTENTS

PART FIVE
ON THE JOB

PART SIX
MANAGING YOUR MONEY

INTRODUCTION

TAKING CONTROL FOR THE NEXT CENTURY

What concerns women most?

This year health is at the top of the list. Actually, health is at or near the top of the list every year. What's new this year is that the topic is heating up. In fact, it's hotter than ever. Only recently the First Congress on Women's Health, held in Washington, D.C., dubbed women's health a major health trend for the twentieth century.

Women doctors and health professionals came to that congress with a strong message: Women feel they've been ignored and short-changed for too long . . . and they've had enough. Women have unique health needs. For years women were routinely left out of medical research projects. They had to plead with their doctors to be taken seriously, then plead for accurate, detailed, intelligent information about their diagnosis and treatment.

Fortunately, that scene is changing fast. In fact, access to health information is *exploding.* For this book we at the Rodale Center for Women's Health have gathered the best information about women's health, written by some of the best popular health writers in the country.

We recognize also that health involves more than physical care. Women have always known that "health" includes the quality of one's relationships with others, financial security, having satisfying, fulfilling work to do, looking good and, in general, feeling good about oneself. *The Healthy Woman* embraces all these subjects.

It's our wish at the Rodale Center for Women's Health and *Prevention* Magazine Health Books that women continue to demand control of their lives—physical, mental and spiritual. It's the healthy thing to do.

Alice Feinstein
Editor

PART ONE

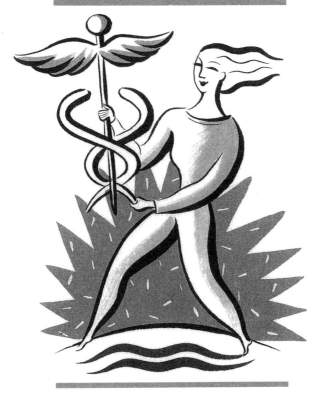

TAKE CONTROL
OF YOUR HEALTH

A NEW ERA
FOR WOMEN'S HEALTH

HERE'S THE LATEST MEDICAL NEWS IN THE 1990S— 25 FINDINGS TO BOOST YOUR HEALTH.

The 1990s are ushering in a new sophistication in women's health. Imagine the discovery of the gene defect that causes breast cancer, which would help doctors prevent the disease in high-risk women. Or skin cancer being prevented with a vitamin-enriched cream, or the symptoms of PMS being reduced with a calcium supplement. And consider: This fantastic voyage is not being driven by the medical establishment alone but also by women themselves, who are more knowledgeable than ever about their own health care.

Below are 25 findings and suggestions from the latest medical information to make this decade your healthiest one yet.

EARLIER DETECTION

1. At least 60 percent of ovarian cancers are detected at advanced stages, when the five-year survival rate is a paltry 5 to 15 percent. Many doctors believe the picture could improve drastically through early detection if women at risk received an annual transvaginal ultrasound test, a painless procedure in which a probe is inserted into the vagina, producing a magnified sonogram of the ovaries and uterus.

Although the ultrasound technique has been used for this purpose for only about two years, it is showing promise in detecting very small tumors long before they can be felt. If you've had breast cancer, you stand twice the chance of developing ovarian cancer and are a good candidate for early screening. Genetic factors are also significant—doctors believe that if a sister, mother or aunt has had ovarian cancer, you're also a candidate, whether you're 20 or 40.

Although federal guidelines have not yet been set, some researchers go further, saying that every woman who's reached menopause should have an annual exam no matter what her perceived risk.

2. Also worth noting is a blood test called the CA 125, which looks for elevated levels of a substance secreted by ovarian tumors. Because the test less accurately detects new tumors than it does recurrences of cancer in the pelvic area, many researchers believe it may work best when used in conjunction with ultrasound. A study is currently under way at the National Cancer Institute to find out.

3. By the end of this decade, nearly two million women will have been diagnosed with breast cancer, and close to 500,000 will die. Many of these lives could be saved if women were to go for periodic mammograms—a baseline by age 35 to 40 and follow-ups every one to two years between ages 40 and 49. The good news: This pricey procedure, which can run as high as $250, is getting easier to pay for, now that 37 states and Washington, D.C., require insurance companies to cover screening mammograms. And more and more companies are offering employees the exams at deeply discounted rates. Either way, statistics show it's worth the investment: Women whose cancers are detected by mammography in the earliest stages have a five-year survival rate of 92 percent, compared with 71 percent or less if the disease has spread past the breast.

4. Colorectal cancer, the third leading cause of cancer mortality in women, affects 77,000 women a year and results in almost 30,000 deaths. To improve survival rates, many doctors now recommend that all women over age 40 get an annual digital rectal exam. Those with a family history of colorectal cancer should start even earlier, and some physicians feel it should be a standard part of an annual physical for all women. The painless exam, which allows the doctor to feel if a tumor is present in the rectum, can be performed at the same time as a pelvic. When colon or rectal cancer is caught early, the five-year survival rate is greater than 80 percent.

PROTECTION FROM THE SUN

5. Women who, despite all the evidence, can't give up tanning should consider using face and body creams laced with vitamin E—though this shouldn't replace the use of sunscreen—because preliminary research shows that these creams may be effective in preventing skin cancer. In a study at the University of Arizona in Tucson, Helen Gensler, Ph.D., found that when a form of vitamin E known as d-alpha tocopherol was applied topically to ultraviolet-exposed mice, their rates of squamous cell cancer decreased by 50 percent. What's more, the mice were ten times more likely than a control group to reject new tumors, indicating that the nutrient may also stimulate the immune system. The vitamin E in most cosmetic creams is in a different form, known as alpha tocopherol acetate, so Dr. Gensler recommends that you look for creams containing d-alpha tocopherol.

6. Sun worshipers often fall prey to small precancerous warts known as actinic keratoses, as well as to the more dangerous basal cell carcinomas. Vitamin A has been shown to reduce these keratoses in animals when used both topically and orally. Now Thomas Moon, Ph.D., also of the University of Arizona, is testing a high-octane vitamin A pill on human subjects. The idea is to see if a mammoth 25,000 international units a day, a dose extrapolated from animal studies, will be safe and effective in humans. While Dr. Moon says that the average person should not consume this much vitamin A daily—severe liver impairment can result—you can do yourself a lot of good right now by meeting the RDA of 5,000 units.

7. One more reason to slather on sunscreen all year round: Your lifetime chance of developing malignant melanoma, the deadliest form of skin cancer, is now 1 in 105. By the year 2000, it will increase to 1 in 70.

LIGHTER EXERCISE

8. Good news for aerobiphobes: A leisurely stroll may be good for your health. In a recent study conducted by the

Cooper Institute for Aerobics Research in Dallas, HDL—or good—cholesterol increased 6 percent whether women walked at a moderate pace (where they were doing about three miles in one hour) or fast (about five miles per hour). This translates to an 18 percent drop in heart disease risk and "supports the argument that simple physical activity is a health promoter," says the institute's research associate, Christopher Scott.

9. What if you don't have your usual 30 to 60 minutes to work out? If you've already achieved a basic level of fitness (exercising three times a week for two to three months), you can temporarily cut back for the next two to three weeks (or longer if you're in very good shape) without sacrificing fitness. Simply shorten your regimen, but stick to your usual intensity. For instance, you can run for 20 minutes instead of 30 as long as you go at your usual speed. Or work out with weights once instead of three times a week, but use the same amount of weight.

10. For couch potatoes who haven't yet gotten the message: Exercising for as little as 30 minutes three times a week may have the same beneficial effect on the heart as quitting smoking.

A NEW LOOK AT WEIGHT LOSS

11. Now that research suggests a link between yo-yo dieting and the risk of heart disease, obesity experts are urging women to rethink dieting—particularly because yo-yo dieting usually leads to weight gain as well. Today's advice: Choose a sensible—rather than an ideal—weight goal. For most women, this means not losing more than 5 percent of your body weight over a three- to six-month period. "By slightly undereating, you'll lose weight more slowly, but you'll no longer be faced with the deprivation that comes from having too little food," says George Blackburn, M.D., Ph.D., of Harvard Medical School in Boston. "And your metabolism will stop working against you."

12. We all know that one of the best ways to lose weight is to cut back on the amount of fat we eat, but no one wants

to eliminate more than she has to. Enter a new program devised by Dr. Blackburn. By cutting your daily fat intake—in grams—to half your weight in pounds, he says, you'll drop the weight and spare yourself the tedious task of calorie counting. If, for instance, you weigh 120, you should not consume more than 60 grams of fat a day.

13. Jean Kristeller, Ph.D., associate professor of psychology at Indiana State University in Terre Haute, has come up with inventive ways for women to enjoy meals without overeating, thus reducing their need to diet. Dr. Kristeller, who began her work at the University of Massachusetts Medical School, teaches the concept of mindfulness, a meditation on food. Here's how to do it: Select a favorite food, say a piece of cake or a cookie. Close your eyes and slowly chew the first bite, paying attention to the sensations it creates on your tongue and as it goes down your throat. Is it hot, cold, moist, scratchy, creamy? When you've finished eating your cake or cookie, notice the effects on your stomach. Through this exercise, explains Dr. Kristeller, "Many women find that the pleasure and fun comes not from six cookies but from one or two eaten with mindful attention."

NUTRIENTS THAT PACK A HEALING PUNCH

14. Including soy products in your diet may help prevent breast cancer. Chemicals known as phytoestrogens, found in those legumes, displace the body's normal estrogens, which may stimulate breast cells and thus lead to cancer. "Phytoestrogens are so weak, they reduce the estrogen stimulation of the breast," says Neal D. Barnard, M.D., president of the Physicians Committee for Responsible Medicine.

Researchers don't yet know how phytoestrogens work after menopause, a time when extra estrogen seems to protect women against osteoporosis.

"One theory holds that it's not the low amount of estrogen after menopause that contributes to osteoporosis but the shift from high estrogen before menopause to low afterward," says Dr. Barnard. "Now we're speculating that it may be more important to lower estrogen through a low-fat diet before menopause rather than boosting it after."

15. New research shows a link between calcium and premenstrual syndrome. In a study conducted at the University of Texas in Galveston and Baylor College of Medicine in Houston, researchers found that women suffering from PMS had significantly lower amounts of calcium in their blood during the luteal—or postovulatory—phase of their cycles. They speculate that calcium may help regulate the release and activity of hormones and have designed a study to determine whether supplementing the diet with calcium will restore levels during that luteal phase. Until results are in, researchers urge all women—especially those suffering from PMS—to meet the RDA for calcium: 1,200 milligrams through age 24, 800 milligrams for women over 25.

16. For some women, a high-carbohydrate, low-fat diet may actually be harmful. According to research by Ann M. Coulston, R.D., at Stanford University Medical Center in California, eating a high-carbohydrate diet may aggravate insulin resistance—a condition where the body's cells become resistant to insulin so the pancreas puts out more and more of it—increasing one's risk of heart disease. Insulin resistance, which affects 10 to 20 percent of the population, may have no symptoms; the condition is only detectable through a special blood test. Who's at risk: anyone who's overweight and sedentary or who has a family history of either diabetes or hypertension.

17. Smokers who meet the RDA for vitamin C may still be suffering from a deficiency, according to a study done at the Medical College of Wisconsin in Milwaukee. Researchers found that smokers needed over 200 milligrams (twice the RDA) of the vitamin to equal the blood levels of nonsmokers consuming 60 milligrams a day. Two eight-ounce glasses of orange juice will make up for the loss.

NEW IDEAS IN REPRODUCTIVE HEALTH

18. Daily low doses of aspirin may hold promise for women who suffer from the leading cause of premature delivery. Preeclampsia, a condition that causes high blood

pressure and severe swelling, affects 5 to 10 percent of pregnant women. A review of six aspirin studies by researchers at Case Western Reserve University School of Medicine in Cleveland found that women who took 1 to 1½ baby aspirin a day during their second and third trimesters reduced their chance of developing pregnancy-induced high blood pressure by 65 percent. And now researchers at more than ten leading medical centers, including the University of Cincinnati, the Medical College of Virginia in Richmond and the University of Pittsburgh, are studying the effects of a daily baby aspirin on this condition. Says Peter VanDorsten, M.D., of the Medical College of Virginia: "What we learn has the potential of making a dramatic impact on the way prenatal care is practiced into the next century."

19. RU 486, the abortion pill, is continuing to show promise for the treatment of endometriosis, an often-painful disorder in which tissue similar to the uterine lining grows outside the uterus. L. Michael Kettel, M.D., of the University of California, San Diego, says 100 milligrams of the drug relieved pelvic pain and reduced endometriotic growths in a small group of patients, although some suffered such temporary side effects as hot flashes, decreased appetite and headaches. Dr. Kettel has since seen similar pain relief at half that dose, and he recently began a study to see if a minuscule 5 milligrams will be equally effective.

20. Another plus for birth control pills: Recent research shows that the risk of endometrial cancer among women who have used the Pill for four or more years is about 60 percent less than it is for women who have never used it.

21. A woman has a 40 percent chance of contracting chlamydia during one act of unprotected intercourse with an infected partner, compared with only a 20 percent chance for a man. This year alone, some 2.5 million women will acquire this sexually transmitted disease. A quarter of them will later suffer from infertility and ectopic pregnancy, the leading cause of pregnancy-related death among black women. Just another reminder: If you're sexually active,

always use a condom. It's your best protection against STDs, including, of course, the AIDS virus.

PROMISING NEW TREATMENTS

22. Doctors believe that giving chemotherapy when tumor cells are dividing most rapidly may make treatments more effective. In research on ovarian cancer patients, Patricia Braly, M.D., associate professor of reproductive medicine at the University of California, San Diego, found that cancer cell activity peaks around noon, while normal cells are most active around midnight. Since most chemotherapy agents target those cells that are dividing the fastest, giving treatments in the morning could zap more of the cancer, she says.

23. Osteoporosis, a thinning of the bones, results in more than 1.3 million fractures and as many as 50,000 deaths each year. The good news: When taken orally, the experimental drug etidronate was shown in clinical trials to significantly increase bone mass in postmenopausal women. After one year of treatment, researchers found a significant decrease in the rate of new bone fractures.

24. Phantom limb syndrome is a well-known complication of amputation, but now the phenomenon is being reported by women who have had their breasts removed by mastectomy. When nerves in the breast are severed during surgery, nerve endings begin to fire abnormally, producing a state of hyperactivity that may lead to phantom pain. This cascade of events can be prevented by injecting local anesthetics into the area before and during surgery, says Mary Ann Ruda, Ph.D., chief of the Section on Cellular and Molecular Mechanisms at the National Institute of Dental Research in Bethesda, Maryland. "This stops the message of pain from getting into the nervous system and helps patients recover more quickly," she says.

25. By the end of the decade, the nation's leading cancer researchers say that they will be able to identify the gene defect responsible for breast cancer, enabling them to replace the faulty protein message and prevent the disease

from developing in women who are at high risk. Says Robert C. Young, M.D., president of Philadelphia's Fox Chase Cancer Center: "The biological control of cancer cells is moving out of the theoretical and into reality."

—*Leslie Laurence*

SIX DISEASES DOCTORS MISS

IF YOUR DOCTOR JUST GAVE YOU A CLEAN BILL OF HEALTH BUT YOU STILL FEEL SOMETHING IS WRONG, YOU COULD BE RIGHT.

One morning Maureen Garcia woke up with a stiff neck, which did not improve after several sessions with her chiropractor. When the pain intensified and spread to Garcia's face, she turned to her family dentist, who treated her unsuccessfully for a jaw disorder called temporo-mandibular joint dysfunction. Finally, after a year of visits to a string of medical specialists and thousands of dollars spent on dead-end tests and treatments, the 38-year-old New York State homemaker was diagnosed with *Lyme disease*—a bacterial infection spread by the bite of a tick.

Garcia's case is not unusual. Recent studies suggest that Lyme disease, as well as several other major illnesses, eludes physicians far more often than you might think. "Medicine is not an exact science," says Michael Fleming, M.D., a family physician in Shreveport, Louisiana, and the spokesperson for the American Academy of Family Medicine. Still, you can get better care if you understand exactly why a diagnosis is so frequently delayed or derailed and if you know how to communicate your symptoms to your doctor. Here's what leading experts say about some commonly misdiagnosed diseases.

QUESTING AFTER ELUSIVE SYMPTOMS

As in Garcia's case, Lyme disease can stump doctors because of its vague symptoms that mimic other ailments. It generally begins with a bout of flulike symptoms, such as fever, headaches, muscle soreness and a stiff neck, which may be followed by facial pain or damage to nerves. Many months into the illness, people often develop arthritis-like joint pain and swelling if the illness is not treated.

Because Lyme disease is relatively rare in many parts of the United States, doctors often blame the early symptoms on more prevalent problems. By the same token, physicians have a tendency to *over*diagnose Lyme in those areas where it's most common, such as the Northeast.

To make matters worse, the blood test for Lyme is often inaccurate. It detects antibodies against the Lyme-causing microbe, but as many as half of those infected do not produce these substances until weeks or months after they become ill, says Robert T. Schoen, M.D., co-director of the Lyme Disease Clinic at the Yale University School of Medicine in New Haven, Connecticut. And a new study found that more than 50 percent of laboratories failed to detect Lyme disease when the level of antibodies was low.

Lack of a reliable test and vague symptoms can also cause doctors to overlook more widespread conditions like *depression*, which affects approximately 15 million Americans. Besides psychological symptoms such as sadness, anxiety and despair, the malady can cause severe insomnia, weight loss, low energy and a diminished sex drive. "There is a tendency to explain away these complaints as a reaction to life events such as marital conflict or aging," says Ari Kiev, M.D., director of the Social Psychiatry Research Institute in New York City.

UPDATING OUTDATED IDEAS

In some cases misinformation can lead doctors down the wrong diagnostic path. Research suggests that some doctors mistake *migraines* for other types of headaches and therefore fail to prescribe specific migraine treatments.

For years physicians have been taught that migraines are always preceded by auras (strange visual images) or numbness, tingling or weakness on one side of the body. But in reality, auras occur in only about one-third of migraine cases. "Despite the 23 million Americans who have migraines, despite the 10 million office visits each year for headaches, most medical school curricula don't contain a lot of information about headache disorders," says Richard B. Lipton, M.D., co-director of the Headache Unit at Montefiore Medical Center in New York City. His new study indicates that 14 million migraine sufferers in this country have never been diagnosed.

Your physician's knowledge may also lag behind current scientific findings in the case of *bacterial vaginosis (BV)*, a vaginal infection that produces a milky discharge and an unpleasant odor. When left untreated, BV—now the leading

HOW TO DISAGREE WITH A DIAGNOSIS

Your doctor has given you a diagnosis and prescribed treatment, but you're not improving as expected. What to do?

You may need a different course of treatment, or the diagnosis may have been incorrect, says family physician Michael Fleming, M.D., of Shreveport, Louisiana, who is spokesperson for the American Academy of Family Medicine. Contact your doctor promptly and give a detailed description of your symptoms, including how long they've lasted.

If several treatments fail and you feel unsure about your condition, it may be time to reevaluate the diagnosis. Don't hesitate to ask your primary-care physician for a referral to a specialist.

If you've seen a specialist and you're still not getting better, get another opinion. Ask your primary-care physician to recommend another doctor, or contact a reputable medical center.

type of vaginal infection in this country—can lead to pelvic inflammatory disease and to preterm labor. Yet many doctors misdiagnose it as a yeast infection, says Jane Schwebke, M.D., medical director of the Chicago Department of Health STD/HIV Prevention Program. Doctors can detect BV with a test that can be done during an office visit.

Misconceptions can even cause *heart disease* to be missed, says Veronica Ravnikar, M.D., a professor of obstetrics and gynecology at the University of Massachusetts Medical Center in Worcester. Although heart disease is the major killer of women over age 50, many doctors fail to see the warning signs—such as unexplained breathlessness, or tightness or pain in the chest—in women because they think of heart disease as a "man's problem," says Dr. Ravnikar. This gender bias may help to explain a disturbing new finding: Two studies found that women are not diagnosed with heart disease until they are more seriously ill than men.

THE NEED TO SCREEN

Sometimes doctors miss a chance for early detection of a deadly disease because they don't suggest screening tests. Experts estimate that deaths from *breast cancer* could be reduced by one-third if all women followed the American Cancer Society's screening guidelines for mammography. Yet studies show that nearly 65 percent of physicians still don't pass on these recommendations to their patients.

Even more shocking is the fact that some breast cancers are missed because the doctor never sees the abnormal mammogram report, warns Janet Osuch, M.D., medical director of the Comprehensive Breast-Health Clinic at Michigan State University in East Lansing. A woman should make sure *she* finds out her test results, says Dr. Osuch.

WHAT YOU CAN DO

A little preparation can help you get a correct diagnosis. When you see your physician, share all your symptoms, even if they seem unrelated. (Dr. Kiev emphasizes the importance of mentioning any changes in your emotional state.) If your doctor orders a test, feel free to ask about its accuracy and the reliability of the lab. And find out the exact diagnosis.

If you have a problem that's hard to pin down, be persistent. "Trust your instincts," says Garcia. "I knew something was wrong—I just didn't know what, and I didn't give up."

—*Susan Chollar*

TAKE THE ACHE
OUT OF BACKACHE

YOU DON'T HAVE TO SUFFER ANYMORE. HERE'S THE LOWDOWN ON HOW TO SOOTHE THE PAIN.

Eight years ago, I became a health statistic. Like four out of five Americans, I suffered a back attack that ultimately would change my life.

Suddenly my back felt made of glass. One wrong move could shatter its delicate equilibrium, sending spasms of agony down my lower back to the toes of my right foot. Years of a sedentary job as a writer, weak back and abdominal muscles and a failure to warm up before exercising made me a prime candidate for a major back incident. The result? A bulging disk pressing mercilessly on my sciatic nerve.

Desperate to recover, I tried virtually every method of pain control. Finally, by learning ways to protect my back during everyday activities—like sitting at my desk—I found relief. Within three weeks, I was back at work and pain free . . . I hope for good.

My experience taught me there's no universal fix for an

aching back. What works for some may not work for others—with one exception. Staying fit—maintaining firm abdominal and back muscles—will help you achieve lifelong flexibility and manage stress, both keys to preventing back problems.

WHY BACKS GO OUT

The spine, an intricate stack of shock-absorbing disks and bony vertebrae, is stabilized by two muscle groups, which help the body lift, straighten and bend forward and control the degree of curvature in the lower back. These muscles, along with posture-supporting muscles in the buttocks and thighs, help us conduct our daily activities without undue strain. But the gradual increase of physical and/or emotional stress to the back over time can trigger muscles to spasm, causing back pain.

Indeed, the likelihood of back pain increases as we age, when spinal disks (ringed by cartilage tissue on the outside and composed of a jellylike center) begin to dehydrate and lose flexibility. Being in poor physical shape, in particular, can aggravate this process and cause a disk to herniate or bulge. "When the back is 'ripe' to go, one awkward movement—bending to pick up something (whether it's light or heavy)—can trigger a back attack," says Diana Long, director of physical therapy at the Texas Back Institute (TBI) in Houston.

THE SELF-HELP SOLUTION

Roughly 75 percent of all back injuries happen after working hours, when we try to compensate for the effects of our stress-filled lives with sporadic exercise or home-improvement projects that our bodies have not been properly conditioned to handle.

Luckily, most of us can survive a back episode without medical help—and resume normal activities in no time. Before you rush off to a doctor, try managing your pain at home.

Stop the pain-producing activity. Avoid lifting your two-year-old or any heavy object. Skip aerobics class and don't sit for long periods of time.

Rest in bed for no more than two days. Until just recently, doctors believed that up to two weeks of bed rest was the best first step to recovery. No longer. New research proves that getting moving soon after a back attack (regardless of whether you still hurt) prevents loss of strength, muscle weakness and ligament tightness, which increase pain.

When you do rest in bed, lie on your back with your knees bent and propped up on one or two pillows, or on your side with a pillow cushioned between your knees. Avoid resting or sleeping on your stomach.

Take aspirin or ibuprofen four times a day. This will help control pain and reduce inflammation the first few days, when the pain is most acute. (Long-term use of pain relievers is not recommended.)

Apply heat, cold or gentle massage. Heating pads, cold packs, over-the-counter ointments and massage (professional or amateur) all can help bring minor back pain under control.

For a homemade cold pack, fill a large zipper-type plastic bag with three parts water and one part alcohol. Freeze to a slush and wrap the bag in a towel.

If pain persists, seek a referral (through your hospital's orthopedics department) to a physiatrist, a physical medicine rehabilitation specialist who can assess nerve function and/or muscle damage by using an arsenal of diagnostic techniques—of which surgery is the very last option. In fact, never allow anyone to rush you to surgery unless a battery of tests (such as x-ray, magnetic resonance imaging or computerized tomography scans) confirms a condition that won't respond to more conservative, noninvasive methods.

WHEN BACK PAIN WON'T GO AWAY

More than 17 million Americans reported chronic back pain in 1990, according to the National Center for Health Statistics in Hyattsville, Maryland. As I know only too well, finding the right help can be a frustrating and all too often unsuccessful endeavor. The correct diagnosis may elude even the best specialists, and you may find yourself spending inordinate amounts of time and money on treatments that ultimately don't work.

But don't give up before you start! With a little trial and error, chances are still very good that you can be helped. Here's a guide to help you.

ONE-STOP SPINE-CARE CENTERS

For a wide array of treatments all under one roof, try the newest option in treating back pain: a visit to one of this country's regional comprehensive spine centers.

There, back pain specialists—from physiatrists and orthopedic surgeons to psychologists and physical therapists—work as a team to solve your back problem once and for all.

Because these centers handle many of the most difficult cases, a hefty 10 to 30 percent of their patients come from out of town. They boast a 90 percent recovery rate—without surgery.

Some of the regional centers include the Texas Back Institute, with offices in Dallas, Houston, Midland and Plano; the San Francisco Spine Institute in Daly City; and the Institute for Low Back Care in Minneapolis, which specializes in treatment of the lumbar spine.

HOW PHYSICAL THERAPY CAN HELP

When Rolando Romo, 45, a community-relations representative from Houston, suddenly became unable to turn his head, he was diagnosed with degenerative arthritis. This condition was causing severe disk deterioration.

Romo's doctor prescribed physical therapy involving lower back and lower neck stretches. Though skeptical, he gave it a try. After just one exercise session, the pain disappeared.

Although considered one of the most effective tools in

combating a back attack, physical therapy should not be undertaken when there's unusual weakness in the extremities, nerve damage or a ruptured disk.

Though many people will, like Romo, improve right away, others may need four to six treatments. Those who don't respond within six visits should be reevaluated. Physical therapy is covered by virtually all insurance carriers.

CAN CHIROPRACTIC HELP?

Recent studies have helped prove the value of chiropractic in treating back pain. For example, in a study published in the *British Medical Journal*, researchers compared the two-year progress of 741 low-back-pain patients treated by either physical therapists performing soft-tissue manipulation or by chiropractors who applied force to their spines to move vertebrae beyond their normal range of motion.

Chiropractic won hands down. While hospital patients began to deteriorate after just six months, chiropractic patients were still doing well two years later.

Chiropractic treatment generally relieves symptoms within six weeks, involving about three treatments per week for the first two weeks, tapering down to once a week or once every other week as the patient improves. Cost varies from $25 to $40 (for a typical 15-minute consultation) and is covered by most insurance policies.

MIND OVER BODY

Registered nurse Jaime Wallace, 34, felt "her life was caving in" and thought she'd have to quit her job when it seemed her back pain would never subside. Then she began treatment at the Pain Management and Behavioral Medicine Center in Farmington, Connecticut. After six months, Wallace learned to recognize stress-triggering events and how to relax her muscles to prevent a pain spasm.

Most back specialists today acknowledge that emotional problems play a role in triggering a back episode. Others believe that back pain is almost always caused by emotional factors.

The guru of this school of thought is John E. Sarno, M.D., professor of clinical rehabilitation medicine at New York University School of Medicine in New York City. Dr. Sarno is convinced that back pain is the brain's way of diverting repressed feelings of anger, anxiety or inferiority to a place where we don't have to deal with them directly—our backs.

Dr. Sarno, who once prescribed two months of physical therapy for back pain, now advises patients to avoid any physical treatments for the back, as they may block recovery. His solution? To teach patients that the pain is acting as a distraction from the underlying emotional problems. His program includes two two-hour lectures, with group follow-up for some patients. Says Dr. Sarno, "The most important factor in recovery is information. It's the 'penicillin' for this disorder."

Just how do you determine which came first—heartache or backache?

IS IT REALLY A BACK PROBLEM?

The following symptoms, alone or when they accompany back pain, warrant immediate medical attention.
- Loss of bowel or bladder control.
- Radiating pain down your arm or leg.
- Numbness or weakness in the hands, arms, buttocks, legs or feet.
- A lump on the spine's surface.
- A dull, aching pain that prevents sleep.
- Back pain that won't subside or that aches in your kidney area.

Such symptoms may indicate any number of underlying problems, from kidney disease to cancer, which have nothing to do with a back problem.

"Ask yourself probing questions about your psychological well-being," advises Arthur White, M.D., medical director of the San Francisco Spine Institute.

Are you under unusual pressure at work or at home? Sudden changes in appetite, sleep, sexual interest, decisiveness or mood—especially feelings of hopelessness and prolonged crying—indicate depression.

Short-term counseling, a brief course of antidepressants (or programs such as Dr. Sarno's) can quickly elevate your mood, control pain and help you deal effectively with difficult people and situations—controlling back pain.

BIOFEEDBACK TO RELAX MUSCLES

Pain management also may involve biofeedback training, a technique that teaches you how to control stress through muscle relaxation. Working with a biofeedback machine, in an average of four to ten 30-minute to one-hour sessions, people may receive feedback on tensions in the muscles and learn to relax them. Home relaxation tapes are also provided.

"Biofeedback helps patients under great stress and others for whom pain has become the dominant event of their lives," says Diane Lokay-Nickell, a behavioral medicine clinician at TBI.

Cost ranges from $50 to $100 per session and is covered by a limited number of insurers. Check with yours first.

LIVING THE GOOD LIFE

A bad back doesn't have to mean a life diminished by disability. You can still remain active as long as you keep back safety in mind. Here are some quick hints.

- Walk instead of jog (for less impact on the spine).
- Swim or bike for cardiovascular fitness and flexibility training.
- Protect your back with a lumbar support when you drive, and move the car seat forward to keep your knees level with your hips. Interrupt long trips with stretch breaks.

- Bend from the knees—not from your waist or back—whenever you pick something up, whether it's light or heavy.
- Practice good posture. Avoid slouching or a "military" position. Tuck in your chin and stomach and move your pelvis slightly forward.
- And don't be afraid to make love. Varying positions to find one good for your back can introduce novelty into your love life and enhance communication.

By following some sensible guidelines, you can live a vigorous, productive, passionate, successful life. I am.

—*Sheila Sobell*

THE HEADACHE HANDBOOK

IF YOU'VE EVER FELT HELPLESS IN THE FACE OF POUNDING HEADACHE PAIN, NOW YOU CAN DO SOMETHING ABOUT IT.

The worst headaches of Eva Legendre's life lasted for almost three years. "I felt as though someone was pounding on my forehead with a baseball bat," says the 47-year-old homemaker from Larose, Louisiana.

Although Legendre had suffered migraines since the sixth grade, she was stunned by the ferocity of the round that struck in late 1987. When her husband drove her to a doctor for pain-relief injections, she was so weak the physician had to come out and treat her in the car.

When the shots didn't work, Legendre consulted dentists, oral surgeons, ophthalmologists and other specialists. One neurologist put her on five different medications. But nothing helped. Legendre vomited so often because of the pain that she became dehydrated and had to be hospitalized twice. "I walked into the hospital with a headache—and walked out with a headache," she recalls.

Finally, a friend told Legendre about the Houston Headache Clinic. Desperate for relief, she and her husband made the five-hour car trip there in February 1990.

Clinic director Ninan Mathew, M.D., a neurologist and chairman of the American Council for Headache Education (ACHE), hospitalized Legendre immediately and treated her with a drug called dihydroergotamine (DHE), which can halt migraines that are already in progress. Dr. Mathew also took Legendre off all the medications she had been taking before, prescribed other preventive drugs, outlined a diet that was low in such common irritants as caffeine and alcohol and gave her biofeedback training.

Within a month, Legendre says, her life was back on track. "I feel like a new person," she declares. "My son says, 'I have my mama back.' "

THE HIGH COST OF HEADACHE

Ten years ago, Legendre's story might not have ended so happily. Since then, however, specialized headache centers have sprung up around the country, and advances in research and an array of drugs have revolutionized treatment. Today, there are medications to prevent severe headaches as well as to stop them. Physicians are learning more about the mechanisms of headaches and have identified a host of factors that can trigger them, and they can help patients reduce the risks through lifestyle changes.

That's welcome news indeed for sufferers of this ailment, the most prevalent pain complaint brought to physicians, according to ACHE. In fact, according to a study at the St. Louis University Medical Center, nearly 38 million Americans experience headaches severe enough to interfere with their daily activities. Headache victims miss more than 157 million workdays annually, costing at least $50 billion in health care and absenteeism.

The emotional costs of headache are high as well.

"Sufferers feel out of control, upset and depressed," says Paul Duckro, Ph.D., associate professor of psychiatry and human behavior at the St. Louis University Medical Center and an expert on headaches. They may also have to cope with their co-workers' and families' disbelief that they can't function when they have "just a headache."

Despite the progress, many Americans continue to believe that little can be done for their headaches. What's more, many physicians remain unaware of all the latest therapies. As a result, most sufferers aren't receiving state-of-the-art treatment. "A dangerous myth about headaches is that you have to live with them," says Dr. Mathew. "But that's simply not true. Between 85 and 90 percent of sufferers can be helped."

UNDERSTANDING DAWNS

Years ago, most scientists thought headaches were caused primarily by muscle tension, or by the dilation and contraction of blood vessels on the surface of and directly beneath the skull, in response to such triggers as stress. Now, however, many doctors believe the explanation is more complex—that changes inside the brain itself are the cause. A number of researchers are focusing on the role of the brain chemical serotonin, which acts on nerves, muscles and blood vessels. "People who are headache-prone seem to have trouble with serotonin regulation," says Dr. Duckro.

Headaches can be triggered by a wide array of factors: chemical, environmental, physical and psychological. Among the most common chemical triggers are alcohol, caffeine, chocolate, MSG, tyramine (an amino acid found in dairy products and organ meats) and the artificial sweetener aspartame (NutraSweet). Some sufferers develop headaches when the weather changes or during physical activities at a high altitude, such as skiing—changes in air pressure are thought to be the trigger. Even having an orgasm can spark a headache, as can bright lights, hunger, smoking and an altered sleep schedule.

Stress can be a trigger for those who are headache-prone. Stress-related headaches can start after the anxiety-producing event is over, when the person finally relaxes.

Experts advise people who have frequent headaches to keep a diary to help them determine which triggers and situations tend to bring on an attack. "Drinking red wine and sleeping late might lead to a headache around the time of the menstrual period, but not necessarily at other times," says Joel R. Saper, M.D., director of the Michigan Head Pain and Neurological Institute in Ann Arbor.

Armed with this increasing body of knowledge, doctors are better able to tailor treatment to each patient's needs.

THE MOST COMMON HEADACHE CULPRITS

Experts divide headaches into two categories. The first, primary headache disorders, are those like migraines, in which the headache itself is the problem.

Secondary headaches are those that are symptoms of other conditions, such as colds, flu, acute sinusitis, eyestrain and exposure to pollutants. (In some cases, headaches can signal life-threatening disorders such as meningitis, brain tumors, blood clots in the brain or even strokes. Such cases are very rare. However, you should seek a doctor's attention immediately to rule out these conditions if a headache is accompanied by fever, stiff neck, loss of speech or paralysis, or if the headache strikes suddenly or pain worsens over days or weeks.)

Below is a listing of the most common types of headache—along with the latest treatment information.

Migraine. Between 8 and 12 million Americans suffer from migraine headaches, about two-thirds of them women; the tendency toward this condition seems to be inherited. During an attack, sufferers feel intense throbbing pain on one or both sides of the head. People who have so-called migraine with aura, or classic migraine, often see colors or flashing lights or suffer temporary vision loss about 15 to 30 minutes before a headache begins. Nausea and vomiting are common. Dizziness and numbness in the face, arm or tongue may also occur, and sufferers often feel exhausted for a day or two after an attack. Migraine without aura, or common migraine, produces the same symptoms but is not preceded by visual or neurological changes.

Some women tend to suffer attacks around their menstrual periods. Researchers attribute this cyclic pattern to the effect of fluctuating estrogen levels on key brain chemicals. According to Dr. Saper, birth control pills can also increase the frequency and severity of migraine attacks, since they also alter estrogen levels.

Doctors can treat migraines in a number of ways. DHE, which Eva Legendre took, and a related medication, ergotamine, have been around for years. But some experts say they are not as widely used as they should be. According to Dr. Mathew, many emergency room physicians still treat migraines with addictive pain relievers such as Demerol. "We are trying to educate doctors to use more specific medications such as DHE instead," he says. "Narcotics don't have any specific effect on the mechanisms that lead to head pain—and people who have frequent migraine attacks can become addicted to them."

Still, the ergotamines are not perfect—they can cause nausea, vomiting and even circulation and cardiac problems. DHE must be delivered by injection. However, doctors are awaiting approval of two advances—a new nasal form of DHE and sumatriptan, a drug that's similar to ergotamine and DHE that can relieve migraine pain within an hour and causes less nausea.

Another important advance is that doctors no longer wait for a migraine to strike to administer relief. Beta blockers and calcium channel blockers—used to treat high blood pressure and heart disease—and a drug called methysergide (Sansert), a serotonin inhibitor, have been found highly effective in preventing migraine. Doctors suspect that they stabilize blood vessels and serotonin levels in the brain. Antidepressants such as amitriptyline (Elavil) and Prozac are often helpful in preventing migraine. In addition, doctors are now testing valproate, a drug used to treat epileptic seizures, for staving off migraine.

Although medication can be very helpful, today's therapeutic options are not limited to the prescription pad. Experts often recommend lifestyle changes that include quitting smoking, sticking to a consistent exercise program and a sensible diet, regular mealtimes and sleep habits, and biofeedback. With biofeedback, people are taught to control aspects of their physiology usually governed by involuntary processes, such as skin temperature; this can abort headache pain.

Tension-type headache. Originally called muscle-contraction headache, it's characterized by pressing, squeezing or aching sensations on the side, front or top of the head or the back of the head and neck. Many experts now believe these headaches result from the same biochemical problems implicated in migraines.

Most people suffer tension headaches only occasionally and can find quick relief with over-the-counter (OTC) pain relievers. There are three kinds: aspirin, acetaminophen and ibuprofen. All the headache relievers on drugstore shelves contain one or more of these, often in preparations that include caffeine, antacids, sedatives and buffering agents. Experts say these medications are effective in nonprescription dosages. "The best way to find the medication that's right for you is through careful trial," says Dr. Saper.

However, it's important not to take painkillers indiscriminately, since each has possible side effects. Unbuffered aspirin and ibuprofen can irritate the stomach. Acetaminophen may cause liver problems in large doses or in small doses in people who already have liver disease. Overuse can backfire, too, ultimately increasing headaches. Researchers speculate that this rebound effect occurs because constant medication may interfere with the brain's own ability to fight pain. If you find yourself using OTC painkillers more than once or twice weekly, you should consider being evaluated by your doctor or even a headache specialist.

Some people do experience chronic tension headache episodes—headaches that occur at least 15 days a month for at least six months. "Sixty to 70 percent of the people who come to headache clinics have chronic daily headaches," says Richard Lipton, M.D., co-director of the headache unit at the Montefiore Medical Center in New York City.

In the past, doctors often prescribed tranquilizers for chronic conditions. Now, however, since doctors regard them as related to migraines, they sometimes treat them with migraine medications and behavior therapies.

Cluster headaches. Marked by piercing pain, almost always on one side of the head in and around the eye, cluster headaches, so called because they occur in groups, each last an average of 45 minutes, while cluster periods can last from 3 to 16 weeks. Cluster headaches can be so agonizing that victims have been known to bash their heads against a wall to try to stifle the pain.

Half a million to two million Americans suffer cluster headaches; most of them are men. Experts suspect that changes in the part of the brain known as the hypothalamus may be partly responsible. They have also found that if a person is in the midst of a cluster period, alcohol can trigger an attack; the pain usually starts immediately after consumption. Smoking may have an effect, too; many sufferers are heavy smokers.

Classic cluster headaches—in which weeks of attacks alternate with periods of remission—are often treated with oxygen inhalation. People can keep a tank in their home or office. When they feel an attack coming on, they can inhale some oxygen and usually prevent the attack. Other mainstays of prevention are steroids, calcium channel blockers, Sansert and lithium.

Surgery is now an option for some people who suffer from long-term cluster headaches. To date, Dr. Mathew and his colleagues have performed the procedure on 75 patients. In this operation—known as radio frequency trigeminal gangliorhizolysis—a needle is inserted through the base of the skull and into the trigeminal nerve, which emerges from the brain, branches out into the facial area and plays a key role in transmitting pain. Electrical currents that can heat and destroy nerve fibers are passed through the needle and kill the pain-carrying fibers of the trigeminal nerve.

"About 75 percent of these people stop having disabling headaches," says Dr. Mathew. But since the surgery can leave parts of the face permanently numb, it is used only in intractable cases.

STILL MORE HEAD POUNDERS

Some less common types of headaches include:

Posttraumatic headache. Researchers report that people who have sustained head or neck injuries, like whiplash or even simple bumps on the head, can experience headache pain that lasts for months or years. "Head and neck trauma probably produce structural or neural changes in the complex computer system of the brain," explains Dr. Mathew. He says that because they have many causes, these headaches are difficult to treat. Doctors often must try various therapies used in other types of headaches before they find one that works.

Sinus headache. Although there are cases in which a chronic sinus infection can trigger the underlying headache process, many people who reach for a decongestant to relieve what they believe is a sinus headache may actually be suffering from migraine or tension headaches. Experts say that actual sinus headaches are associated with colds, sneezing, a runny nose or hay fever.

TMJ headaches. Some people attribute their headaches to temporomandibular joint (TMJ) syndrome, a dysfunction of the temporomandibular joint, one of the two joints connecting the lower jawbone to the skull. While TMJ pain can trigger the headache process in some cases, doctors now believe many such people may actually be migraine victims. "TMJ problems can cause facial pain, but they rarely cause recurrent, severe headaches," says Dr. Mathew. "A lot of people with migraines undergo unnecessary, expensive surgery to the temporomandibular joint and end up with the same headache."

HAPPY ENDINGS

As for Legendre, she is now almost headache free—and doing everything she can to stay that way. Upon her release from the hospital, she had strict instructions to stay away from her particular triggers: cheese, caffeine, aspartame and preservatives. She now eats three balanced meals a day, or six mini-meals. She also does aerobic exercise at least three times a week, walks a mile each day and listens to a biofeedback tape regularly to ease stress.

She's had one flare-up, but a short-term regimen of Prozac got her back on track. Now when she feels a twinge of discomfort, perhaps once a week, Legendre takes Midrin—a capsule containing acetaminophen, a sedative and a blood vessel dilator—and lies down for a while. Her husband, Earl, can also administer DHE injections in emergencies. So far, this regimen seems to be working. "I can't believe the difference," she says.

Legendre has resumed the housework and gardening she gave up when her daily headaches disabled her. Reports her husband, "She's back to her normal self."

—*Saralie Faivelson*

STAYING WELL IN A SICK BUILDING

WHAT TO DO WHEN YOUR HEADACHE AND SNIFFLES DISAPPEAR MIRACULOUSLY EVERY AFTERNOON AT PRECISELY 5 P.M.

If tissues are the most coveted supply in your office and "the bug" seems to have established permanent residence, the problem could be your building, not the people in it.

Poor indoor air quality (IAQ) is now considered one of the nation's leading environmental health threats. Industry experts estimate that between 20 and 30 percent of all non-industrial buildings have indoor air pollution levels high enough to give 20 to 50 million of the people working in them flu- and allergy-like symptoms. And if each employee suffering from poor IAQ loses six minutes of concentration ability a day—the equivalent of three sick days a year—the indirect cost to employers is $10 billion annually.

Alice Farrar is a certified industrial hygienist and vice president of quality management and marketing at the Atlanta office of Clayton Environmental Consultants, one of the largest and oldest of the environmental consulting firms. Its client list includes the Occupational Safety and Health Administration (OSHA) and the Environmental Protection Agency (EPA). Here's how Farrar answers questions about the problem of workplace air pollution.

Q: **Why is indoor air quality such a concern today?**

A: During the energy crisis of the 1970s, we started building high-rise office buildings with sealed windows because they could be heated and cooled more efficiently. Unfortunately, the ventilation systems in these "tight" buildings are often poorly designed or maintained. It's not just a matter of a few people complaining about tobacco smoke or the temperature. Poor IAQ can cause headaches and fatigue, making it difficult to concentrate and thereby decreasing productivity. In extreme cases, IAQ problems can result in Legionnaires' disease, asthma, even cancer.

Q: **What is sick-building syndrome (SBS)?**

A: We diagnose a building as being "sick" when more than 20 percent of the people working in it complain of headaches, dizzy spells, sore throats, itchy eyes, nausea, skin irritations or coughs, and when workers get better 12 to 24 hours after leaving the building. Some people whose respiratory systems have become infected with minute particles of bacteria or fungi, called microbiologicals, stay sick.

Q: What causes SBS?

A: A poorly designed ventilation system is the major culprit. Buildings need a source of fresh air to disperse odors and fumes, but many ventilation systems have the outdoor-air intake right next to the exhaust vents coming from the restrooms, kitchens or chemistry labs. That means their own contaminants are drawn back in. To eliminate cross-contamination, either the intake or the exhaust needs to be moved, which can be a major undertaking. Another problem is that many ventilation systems aren't regularly cleaned or switched on. You can also track down the sources of the contamination and remove them.

Q: What are some of the major indoor air pollutants?

A: Tobacco smoke is a big one, as well as fumes from building materials and furnishings. Most wall coverings, paint, glue and cloth-covered office-space dividers will give off volatile organic compounds (VOCs), toxic vapors or gases when they're new. Fax and copy machines give off VOCs while they're in use. Maintenance people also like to put insecticide in the heating units along office walls or windows. The air passing through spreads these chemical poisons into the office. Another problem is airborne microbiologicals, which can grow on any wet surface as an orange or green mold, in the drain pans or ducts of the ventilation system or anyplace there's been water damage.

Q: Can VOC levels be controlled?

A: If the contaminant levels are moderate and the ventilation system is good, the VOCs will eventually dissipate. In a typical building, this takes from three to six months. In poorly ventilated buildings, the levels can stay high enough to irritate for up to a year or more. That's why it's a good idea for IAQ experts to be involved in designing a building.

Q: **What can individuals do to alleviate SBS symptoms?**

A: A short-term solution would be to move your seat if you're sitting near or under an air register. If you must use a humidifier or dehumidifier, change the water daily—microbiologicals can grow in the old water. You might feel better putting a small fan in your office, but a fan is a sign of a problem, not a solution. And while plants won't hurt, they're not clean-air machines.

You should also talk to your peers and your supervisor to see if they're experiencing any symptoms. Keep track of health complaints, show your record to personnel and suggest they have the building manager get "Building Air Quality," a booklet put out by the EPA and the National Institute for Occupational Safety and Health.

—Linda J. Murray

A NEW VIEW OF YOUR MENSTRUAL CYCLE

YOUR MENSTRUAL CYCLE CAN BE A POSITIVE MIND/BODY EXPERIENCE THAT INFLUENCES CREATIVITY AND SEXUAL DESIRE.

Memories of my first period are strong. My blood began flowing shortly after my 12th birthday. Everyone around me, I was sure, could smell me. I felt opened up, exposed, convinced the blood was pouring out by the pint.

The term *sexuality* wasn't part of my vocabulary at such an age, but with my first period I suddenly felt sexual: sexually vulnerable, sexually aware and sexually embarrassed. Etched in my mind is the day I wore the same pad during a full day of school. I laugh about it now, but back then I feared that the older girls hanging out in the bathroom would make fun of me if they saw me carrying my soiled pad from the stall to the trash can.

In the months afterward, my relationships with boys changed. They became the capable, the powerful, while I gradually felt less capable, less powerful, with a bulky pad hampering my activities. Slowly, the tomboy in me disappeared.

I'm recalling this story because it's likely that millions of other American women had a similar sort of experience with their first period. It's probably hardly necessary to say that most women view their periods as a messy and unfortunate biological monthly inconvenience. But why do we think of menstruation in this way?

"The truth is that [first] menstruation . . . points us inexorably forward into womanhood [while] at the same time it turns us back, regressing us in its own unheeding manner to that earlier time when we were unable to control our bodies," writes Nancy Friday in her ground-breaking 1977 book, *My Mother, My Self.*

GETTING A NEW VIEW

However, the current thinking on the subject by some feminist doctors, health-care specialists, psychologists and academics is that there's a new sensibility emerging among women about their menses. It involves learning to reenvision menstruation, indeed the entire menstrual cycle, as a symbol of our feminine power—a time of heightened creativity, intuition and insight. This is an important developmental step, say the experts, for without it we may be destined to carry a negative attitude about our cycle throughout adulthood.

Of course women aren't born with bad feelings about our bodies. Many others "help" us in this respect. Although there are many men, for instance, who are sympathetic toward their partner's distress both premenstrually and during her periods, there are others for whom this is an uncomfortable subject.

"What creates men's anxiety [about menstruation] is not only that it is a mystery connected with the female anatomy," says Richard Robertiello, M.D., in *My Mother, My Self.* "It is also a reminder of another feminine mystery . . . the power to reproduce. Men don't have this power, so it makes them edgy." Menstruation may also unconsciously remind men of the time when a woman was "all-powerful in every man's life," says Dr. Robertiello, " . . . when he was a baby. . . . Do you think those humiliations are all forgotten? Not in the subconscious, they're not."

SURROUNDED BY PUT-DOWN

Because society has traditionally viewed female sexuality—including the menstrual cycle—as both shameful and insignificant, negative attitudes toward menstruation are held by women as well as men. For example, preliminary research indicates that a sizable minority of both sexes believe the old myth that women cannot function normally while menstruating. In a 1981 study of 1,034 women and men conducted by the Tampax Corporation, a third of the male respondents and one-fourth of the females agreed with the statement that women do not function as well at work during menstruation as they do when not menstruating.

And alas, because many of our mothers were raised to feel ashamed of their bodies and cycles, they unconsciously passed those same messages on to us.

Advertising plays its part, too. TV commercials, for example, encourage women to devalue menstruation by rarely, if ever, acknowledging that we're dealing with women's menstruation, our *blood.* Instead we are urged to hide "that time of the month" while maintaining our "confidence."

Many doctors also perpetuate our discomfort with menstruation. They tend to focus our attention on the problematic aspects of our cycles—especially premenstrual syndrome, or PMS (the cluster of symptoms, which include cramping, depression, bloating, anxiety and irritability, among others, that many women experience in the week before their periods). As a result, the majority of women focus on the pains of PMS and the inconvenience of menstruation rather than seeing what Bethany Hays, M.D.—an obstetrician/gynecologist at Women to Women, a women's health center in Yarmouth, Maine—calls the "serious magic" of the menstrual cycle, PMS and all.

THE FEMALE CYCLE AS MAGIC

"Imagine a being that bleeds but is not wounded. Imagine a being that bleeds but does not die. Is it a magical, mythical creature, or merely a woman? Or both? Can such a being be 'merely' woman? There is a certain mystery here, of which man can know nothing, and women must know something," writes Barbara Black Koltuv, Ph.D., in *Weaving Woman: Essays in Feminine Psychology from the Notebooks of a Jungian Analyst.* Reenvisioning the female cycle involves an appreciation of the blood mysteries—menstruation, pregnancy/birth, menopause—Dr. Koltuv writes about. Matriarchal cultures, says Dr. Koltuv, concerned themselves with fertility and nature, which were honored through rites and myths. The phases of the moon were believed to be intimately connected to women's nature.

"We are [still] cyclic," says Dr. Hays, "like the moon. The moon is symbolic of our menstrual cycles." Even the length of a woman's cycle corresponds to that of the moon's—about 29½ days. Our cycles, writes Dr. Koltuv, "consist of change, process, and transformation . . . .This is the miraculous, transformative aspect of women . . . affecting our energy, our [ideas], our emotions, and [it] is the matrix of our very nature."

Indeed, the moon does seem to reflect the birth-and-death cycle going on inside of women during the menstrual cycle. The bright orb of the full moon is like the egg we release at ovulation. The dark moon is like the death of the orb, like the shedding of our blood where the egg would have grown had conception occurred. Dr. Hays believes that it is this cycle of death and rebirth of the moon—a creation and re-creation—that is embodied in a woman, allowing her not only to create life in the form of a child but to re-create herself as she evolves emotionally, professionally and spiritually.

When women become aware of the connection between their own cycles and those of the moon, we can begin to appreciate our deep interconnection with the natural world—a fact all too easy to forget in the stress-ridden, technology-filled lives most of us lead. According to Dr. Hays: "When you believe your period is a symbol of your power, your ability to give birth and the magical mysterious qualities of being a woman, this increases your ability to get in touch with the [shifts in] intuition, creativity and emotions you experience during your cycle. You begin to accept and sometimes even look forward to your period."

EASING THE PAIN

Viewing our menstrual cycles as a symbol of female strength can actually lessen the physical and emotional discomfort of PMS for some women, since our minds have a profound effect on our bodies, and vice versa. Dr. Hays explains: "The brain is connected to different parts of the body via chemical messengers that float in the bloodstream and 'communicate' with all the organs, including the uterus and ovaries, through receptors in those organs."

Therefore, if we feel negatively about our female organs or menstruation, says Dr. Hays, we may experience PMS symptoms such as cramping and headaches as more painful. This is not to say that women are to blame for painful PMS symptoms; we're not. But if we think positively about our cycles, those symptoms will often be easier to tolerate, says Dr. Hays.

CREATIVITY DURING THE CYCLE

Just as the mind affects the body, the body also affects the mind. In fact, some physicians and scientists theorize that "women go through an identifiable and observable series of consciousness shifts as they travel through their hormonal cycle," says Tamara Slayton, director of the Menstrual Health Foundation, a nonprofit educational center in Sebastopol, California. We can get in touch with these consciousness shifts by listening carefully to the signals that our minds and bodies send us. Here are some of the latest theories about the female cycle.

During the beginning of the cycle, there is a rise in estrogen, a buildup of tissue in the womb and an increased blood supply to the uterus. At this time, writes feminist author Demetra George in *Mysteries of the Dark Moon: The Healing Power of the Dark Goddess*, "women feel more energetic, optimistic and emotionally expansive. This is a powerful time; women can use this energy high by taking risks" or putting plans into action.

Around the time of ovulation, when estrogen levels peak, Dr. Hays believes that creativity may be at its peak for some women. (Other women may find this occurs at other times of the month.) This creativity isn't just limited to artistic expression, she says. "For some women, creativity is coming up with great ideas, for some it's the ability to think of new recipes, while for others it's getting flashes of insight about their lives. It depends on each woman's definition of creativity."

The cycle nears its end in the two weeks before menstruation, as hormone levels begin to fall (provided conception has not occurred). Moodiness and irritability, two classic premenstrual symptoms, often occur during this time. However, according to Lara Owen, author of *Her Blood Is*

MOODY, AND PROUD OF IT

More than one woman with PMS has been described as a moody bitch. But Tamara Slayton, director of the Menstrual Health Foundation, a nonprofit educational center in Sebastopol, California, has redefined the term to help women recognize that there could be a method to their madness. "BITCH," says Slayton, is an acronym for Being In Touch Creates Havoc. When you no longer censor your angry or sad feelings—when you no longer put other people's feelings first, as many women do much of the time—people may be shocked. But expressing your emotions is a healthy release, as long as you don't verbally abuse others.

Gold: Celebrating the Power of Menstruation, this emotionality is a kind of psychological safety valve that promotes a healthy self-awareness.

"Many women lead pretty impossible lives these days—women who have families and jobs and who then come home and take care of everyone else," says Owen. "PMS may be a way of expressing the pent-up anger we feel over not having any time to ourselves." Of course, each woman will communicate her anger differently: Some are cranky, while others experience sadness. It's important to realize that these are not new "crazy" feelings brought about by our hormones; instead, we're simply bringing our real hidden emotions to the surface.

During menstruation—the end of the cycle—progesterone and estrogen are at their lowest levels. The blood and uterine lining that were being built up in the first half of the cycle are now being expelled from the body. At this time, writes George, "a woman turns inward emotionally and physically." According to Dr. Hays, women also tend to feel their calmest at this point. Menstruation is also a time, says George, when a woman may intuitively want to clear her psyche, as her body is cleansing the uterus.

"This is a prime time for her to engage in all kinds of inner work," according to George, such as focusing in on what she's doing with her life. On a clearly practical level, Dr. Koltuv says: "Have you ever just stood in front of the refrigerator and started throwing away all the leftovers, all the jars of stuff you haven't used in months, while in the background your husband complains that you're crazy? Notice if this happens during your period. It's the everyday side of cleansing your life in the way your uterus is cleansing itself."

MENSTRUATION AND SEX

Sex during our periods is generally considered taboo. Besides the fact that many men are turned off by the idea, "a lot of women have picked up the idea that sex during this time is unclean," says Dr. Hays—something that "nice" women don't desire.

In fact, sex during menstruation is a pleasurable experience for many women. "Many researchers have shown that there are rises in sexuality during the course of the menstrual cycle," say Penelope Shuttle and Peter Redgrove in their book *The Wise Wound: The Myths, Realities and Meanings of Menstruation.* "Some . . . have found that the chief rise is during the four days before your period and the four days after it has begun."

There may be a physiological reason for this: Orgasm during menstruation can relieve cramping. Says Dr. Hays: "Although there are many women who are not particularly interested in vigorous sex during their period, sexual excitement does produce tremendous changes in blood supply and a release of endorphins [chemicals associated with a sense of well-being] that may give some women relief from cramping."

RIDING THE CYCLES OF LIFE

Women who start to pay attention to their cycles and honor the different emotional, creative and sexual changes they undergo each month "have far fewer problems during their cycle," argues Dr. Koltuv. Acceptance of your cycle isn't a passive experience. Rather, it's a cognitive process of listening to the wisdom of your body and following its clues—for sleep, for expression, for sexual union, for solitude, for creating your life's path.

In addition to paying more careful attention to our cycles, proper diet and exercise are, of course, also necessary for what Slayton refers to as menstrual health. "It is impossible to overestimate the importance of good nutrition in controlling PMS," says Susan M. Lark, M.D., in her *Premenstrual Syndrome Self-Help Book.* Dr. Lark, who is the director of the PMS and Menopause Self-Help Center in Los Altos, California, believes that "no medication can entirely overcome the effects of a poor diet."

She recommends that women eat a healthful, natural diet, which includes foods such as whole-grain cereals, whole-grain breads, beans, vegetables, fish and lean poultry, fruits, nuts and seeds. She advises women to avoid "coffee, cola drinks, candy, cookies and ice cream. These foods can disrupt your hormonal chemistry."

Dr. Lark also recommends exercise as a way of relieving the anxiety and irritability of PMS. It can help relieve bloating and backache as well, she says.

If we want to have a more stress-free, comfortable, pleasant menstrual cycle, Dr. Lark believes that we must honor it first. Honoring our bodies leads to accepting them as they are. Once we accept and value our cycle as a natural part of being female, we can reclaim what has been lost to us for so many years. For to reclaim our cycles is to revere the powers—intuitive, creative, sexual—residing deep within all women.

—*Lisa Couturier*

IN SEARCH OF A GOOD NIGHT'S SLEEP

DRUGS ARE OUT, HERBS ARE IN, AND DOCTORS ARE TELLING SLEEPLESS PEOPLE TO DO ANYTHING—EXCEPT TRY TOO HARD.

At cocktail parties and on coffee breaks, people trade insomnia cures like cookie recipes. "Try this," someone says, proffering a blister pack of Quiétude tablets, a handful of valerian capsules or the name of an acupuncturist penciled on the back of a business card.

One out of three people suffers bouts of sleeplessness that may last a few nights or a few weeks, according to the National Sleep Foundation. But enlightened people, with their doctors' support, are more inclined to try natural approaches than sleeping pills.

"I feel desperate when I have insomnia," one New York woman confides, "but I won't take drugs. That would be crossing the line." She finds hot baths and a cup of Sleepytime tea comforting. And many doctors now would rather search for a cause than cover a symptom. Treating lack of sleep with sleeping pills, says Peter Hauri, Ph.D., a clinical psychologist and administrative director of the Mayo Clinic Sleep Disorders Center in Rochester, Minnesota, is tantamount to prescribing painkillers without bothering to find the pain's source.

Everyone talks about insomnia, though two people rarely mean the same thing when they use the word. Insomnia, a vague term that describes a symptom more than it defines a syndrome, is a vicious cycle of sleeplessness and sleepiness that undermines the quality of a person's life. (Sharks never sleep, and we all know how nasty they are.)

"Insomnia may arise from psychological issues such as anxiety or depression, medical problems, a lifestyle that invites lots of jet lag, or poor sleep habits," explains Dr. Hauri.

HELP FOR THE SLEEPLESS

To help those who continually have trouble either falling or staying asleep or those who struggle through each day because their nightly rest is not restorative, diagnostic expertise is available at accredited sleep labs. The number of accredited sleep disorder centers in the United States has risen from 3 in 1978 to more than 200 in 1992.

Some people with insomnia pay up to $1,000 a night to bed down at one of these places, with electrodes pasted on their heads and over their hearts to measure the physiology of their sleep states. But most sleep center treatments are provided on an outpatient basis, with people calling or dropping in at the center periodically for advice, encouragement or, in extreme cases, prescription medicines.

A Gallup Organization poll commissioned by the National Sleep Foundation found that despite the proliferation of sleep clinics, the majority of the nation's 35 million self-proclaimed insomniacs shun medical treatment. Unaware that professional help is available or embarrassed to discuss their condition with their doctors, they often medicate themselves with "inappropriate remedies" that fail, says former foundation president Thomas Roth, Ph.D.

"I picture people awake in the middle of the night, thinking the rest of the world is asleep, and rummaging around their houses looking for anything they can find that may help," says psychologist Mark Chambers, Ph.D., of the Stanford University Medical Center Sleep Disorders Clinic in California. "People who come to our center have tried everything else first. They've done hypnosis and biofeedback. They've sniffed glue and drunk vanilla extract."

According to the Gallup Organization results, alcohol, the proverbial nightcap, remains one of the most widely used home remedies for insomnia. "Alcohol is the world's oldest sleeping pill because it works initially," concedes psychiatrist Quentin Regestein, Ph.D., director of the Sleep Clinic at Brigham and Women's Hospital in Boston.

"The problem is, in the middle of the night, it works the other way." Dr. Regestein says that the effects of alcohol wear off in a few hours and may cause the later stages of sleep to unravel into frequent arousals and difficulty getting back to sleep. This, too, is insomnia. Many women at sleep clinics are surprised to find that just forgoing their daily drink at dinner or bedtime is all they really need to do to eliminate their sleep problems, says Dr. Chambers.

SLEEPING BETTER WITH HERBS

On the national level, over-the-counter sleep aids advertised on television (many of which contain antihistamines that induce drowsiness) are just ahead of alcohol in popularity. But the more sophisticated and adventurous sleep-deprived prefer exotic soporifics. In Los Angeles, for example, numerous movie stars and models receive a mix of acupuncture and herbs from Drew Francis, an acupuncturist and a doctor of Oriental medicine. At the Golden Cabinet, Francis's clinic/apothecary, he treats 10 to 20 clients each week for complaints related to insomnia.

For chronic insomnia, Francis prescribes a ten-treatment course of acupuncture (or acupressure for the needle shy), augmented with exercise, relaxation and individually tailored herbal formulas. Ziziphus, an herb with strong soporific effects, figures as a key ingredient in Francis's popular "Heavenly Emperor's Tonify the Heart Decoction." Ginseng, coptis, angelica and longan are other herbs Francis prescribes in combination to help people achieve a more balanced state—with more mental alertness during the day and better sleep at night. Occasionally he prescribes a nighttime-only formula called Jinbuhuan (translated as "more precious than gold"), a heavy-duty insomnia treatment for people who have tried other formulas without success.

Western medicine also has an herbal tradition, and time-honored substances such as valerian are gaining popularity as the accelerated pace of life makes slowing down to sleep harder. This dried root is said to smell like dirty socks, but powdered valerian is available in capsules, often mixed with other herbal sedatives like passionflower and hops.

"To my great surprise, valerian has shown itself to be effective in European clinical trails," says Dr. Hauri, who is the author, with Shirley Linde, of *No More Sleepless Nights*. Dr. Hauri tells his patients to try valerian if they think it might help, but to do so scientifically, experimenting for at least a week and keeping written records of how they sleep each night. Herbalists who praise valerian's virtues caution that continued use of high dosages can bring on anything from headaches and heart disturbances to aggravated insomnia.

Another alternative is the homeopathic insomnia remedy called Quiétude, which has been sold in France for 20 years under the name Sedatif PC. Quiétude contains infinitesimal amounts of plant extracts, including belladonna and calendula, that are commonly thought to reduce stress and tension.

SLEEP RIGHT, SLEEP BETTER

Sleep experts are heading a trend away from prolonged use of sleep medications of any kind—for the simple reason that the drugs don't work in the long run. Several published studies have shown not only that sleeping pills fail to improve the quality of sleep but also that withdrawal of the drugs results in "rebound insomnia," which leaves sleep-troubled people worse off than before. Informed physicians prescribe such drugs judiciously and for very brief periods—to help a person get some rest during a profound personal crisis, for instance.

A better approach to the problem of insomnia, improbable as it sounds, may be to restrict the amount of time a person spends in bed. Wolfgang Schmidt-Nowara, M.D., director of the University Hospital Sleep Center in Albuquerque, New Mexico, recently completed a three-year clinical trial based on this theory.

"Many people who have insomnia spend too much time in bed as part of their desperate attempt to get more sleep," Dr. Schmidt-Nowara says. They hasten to bed early, worried about the time it will take them to fall asleep. And when they awaken, they lie in bed as long as possible, anxious and overtired, hoping to fall asleep again. The idea behind sleep-restriction therapy, which was developed by psychologist Arthur Spielman, Ph.D., director of the Sleep Disorders Center of the City College of New York, is to cut out the wasted hours.

In a New Mexico sleep-restriction study, for example, subjects were asked to keep sleep logs for several weeks, and then each person was given a strict limit on time in bed. "When we told people who were used to nine or ten hours a night that they could have only six, they panicked," recalls study nurse Carol Jessop, R.N. About three-quarters of the subjects experienced dramatic relief from insomnia. "The ones who responded began to sleep all or most of the time they were in bed, and then they saw for the first time that something was going to work for them."

Scientists are also studying whether exercise can reduce sleeplessness. "The idea that a good workout promotes good sleep is practically a truism," says Dr. Chambers. "But there's been no research to confirm the idea among people with insomnia." Postexercise fatigue, Dr. Chambers points out, is not the same phenomenon as brain sleepiness. What's more, exercise performed very late in the day may prove overstimulating and sleep-defeating. He believes well-timed exercise will eventually be proven beneficial.

"The key element is to raise the body temperature," Dr. Chambers explains. Exercise that significantly increases body temperature, followed by a cooling-down period of a few hours, may help relieve insomnia because it mimics that natural drop in body temperature that presages the onset of sleepiness at night. Dr. Chambers adds that a hot bath toward bedtime might accomplish the same end.

Many sleep experts are convinced that the back-to-basics approach may be the healthiest solution: Establish a nightly routine that brings on tiredness. If a hot bath and a glass of warm milk don't do it, get up and read a good book. You'll sleep better tomorrow.

—*Dava Sobel*

THE TEN MOST IMPORTANT HEALTH QUESTIONS YOU CAN ASK

ARMED WITH THE RIGHT INFORMATION, YOU CAN TAKE CHARGE OF YOUR OWN HEALTH CARE.

Most of us value our health—yet the pursuit of a healthy lifestyle often seems too time-consuming a chore. It doesn't have to be. You can maximize your health without committing major amounts of time, if you know where to focus your efforts. To help you jump-start a personal program, a wide range of medical experts answers the ten most important health questions for young women. Here are their commonsense solutions you can implement today.

Q: **1. How critical to my health is my family's medical background?**

A: "Most health problems arise because of a genetic predisposition," says Vivian Terkel, M.D., associate clinical professor of medicine at the University of California, San Diego. For this reason, you need to examine your family's medical history at least as far back as your grandparents to discern patterns of disease inheritance. Pay close attention to diseases affecting your parents and siblings; those are the ones to which you may be most susceptible.

Find out about any chronic diseases, as well as how long each family member lived and the cause of his or her death. Be on the alert for breast and ovarian cancers, especially if a close female relative suffered from either before menopause, says Dr. Terkel. And don't neglect colon cancer. If either of your parents has had multiple polyps of the colon—which, left untreated, develop into cancer—you have a 50 percent risk of being affected, says Aubrey Milunsky, M.D., director of the Center for Human Genetics at Boston University School of Medicine. Also ask about such conditions as high blood pressure, mental illness, alcoholism and multiple miscarriages, all of which may have a genetic component.

Whether or not you find anything suspicious in your family background, you still should see an internist to "go through your family history and come up with a preventive plan for the rest of your life," says Dr. Terkel. If you are vulnerable to a particular condition, you may be able to beat the odds by taking precautions—in the case of heart disease, for example, by controlling your weight, blood pressure and cholesterol and by not smoking. You can also take advantage of early detection. According to Dr. Terkel, your internist can give you guidelines, "but the general rule of thumb with regard to breast cancer, for example, is to start getting annual mammograms ten years before the age that a mother or first-degree relative developed the disease."

In some cases, a visit to a geneticist can eliminate or confirm your concerns. For example, genetic tests can tell you whether you are predisposed to a handful of disorders, such as muscular dystrophy, and whether you are a gene carrier for other diseases, including cystic fibrosis. Knowing that you have not inherited a gene can ease your mind considerably, but there are some caveats. The tests can be expensive—it can cost as much as $500 just to test for muscular dystrophy, for example. And while some private insurers cover these tests, geneticists warn that a positive result can subject you to not only psychological but also social and financial consequences—such as job discrimination and loss of health insurance. For these reasons, it's important to discuss with your doctor the pros and cons of confirming a hereditary disease.

Whatever your family history, keep in mind that "there are very few genetic conditions where we can say it's certain you will get the disease," says Steven Shea, M.D., associate professor of medicine and epidemiology at the Columbia–Presbyterian Medical Center in New York City. "Family history should be a cause for alertness, not alarm."

Q: **2. What is the most important dietary change I can make?**

A: If you guessed eating a low-fat diet (i.e., restricting fat to less than 30 percent of total calories), you're right—with this proviso: Instead of obsessing about the fat content of every item on your plate, says Wayne Callaway, M.D., associate clinical professor at George Washington University Medical School in Washington, D.C., focus on your total fat intake over several days or a week, then make sensible trade-offs. "Permanently forbidding yourself certain foods isn't a very effective long-term strategy for behavioral change," says Dr. Callaway. So you can have sausage for breakfast, as long as you go easy the next day by eating foods low in fat. If you feel you need more of a regimen, limit yourself to one or two servings of fatty foods a day, says Jodie Shield, R.D., a national spokesperson for the American Dietetic Association.

Q: 3. How can I best preserve my fertility?

A: Contraception, lifestyle choices and reproductive disorders may all affect a woman's ability to conceive. Most methods of birth control do not endanger fertility. The most notorious example of one that did was the old Dalkon Shield, an IUD that was linked to pelvic infection in some women, says Russell Malinak, M.D., director of the Center for Reproductive Medicine and Surgery at the Methodist Hospital of Baylor College of Medicine in Houston.

Today, however, there are two new IUDs on the market that are considered much safer. Although some doctors are still hesitant to give the IUD to women who have not yet started or completed their families, Dr. Malinak says that for women in monogamous relationships, because they are less likely to be exposed to sexually transmitted diseases (STDs), the IUD isn't likely to harm fertility. But doctors believe that women who have borne children are better IUD candidates because their uteruses are less likely to expel the device.

Women who have multiple sexual partners should avoid the IUD and always use a condom, even if they're also using another method of birth control. Besides offering substantial protection from the AIDS virus, condoms help prevent STDs such as gonorrhea and chlamydia, which can cause damage to the fallopian tubes and lead to a future ectopic pregnancy or infertility.

If you have a reproductive disorder that could interfere with fertility—including endometriosis and possibly fibroids—your doctor may recommend surgery. To preserve fertility, "make sure the surgery is performed by a reproductive endocrinologist or infertility specialist," says Florence

Haseltine, M.D., Ph.D., an obstetrician/gynecologist with the National Institutes of Health in Bethesda, Maryland. "She'll use smaller stitches and more meticulous surgical techniques to prevent adhesions, tissue formations that may stop the egg from getting to the tube."

Q: **4. No matter how hard I try, I can't stick to a regular exercise program. What is the minimum I need to do?**

A: Fortunately, it takes a lot less activity than most of us think to get significant health benefits—that is, a decreased risk of heart disease, cancer and osteoporosis, plus help with weight control. According to a report published in the *Annual Review of Public Health*, a minimum of 30 minutes of daily physical activity, even at a moderate pace, will confer these benefits, says principal author Steven Blair, P.E.D. (doctor of physical education), director of epidemiology at the Cooper Institute for Aerobics Research in Dallas. Some studies even suggest that as little as 15 to 20 minutes a day may be enough to promote health.

Exercises that qualify include such relatively lightweight activities as pleasure bicycling, gardening, housework and making love, says James Rippe, M.D., director of the Exercise, Physiology and Nutrition Laboratory at the University of Massachusetts Medical School in Amherst. Specialists call this approach "lifestyle exercise as opposed to planned formal exercise," says Dr. Blair, author of *Living with Exercise*. That means, for example, that if you hate going to the gym but love being outdoors, you can turn the chore of taking out your dog into an enjoyable 20-minute walk before or after work. "It's not as if you're either a slug or an athlete," says Dr. Blair. "There's a whole spectrum in between."

To reinforce your commitment, try adding mental imagery to your activity. A study conducted by Dr. Rippe and Ruth Stricker, who develops mind/body principles for exercisers, found that using cognitive strategies such as deep breathing during low-intensity walking significantly reduced anxiety and improved self-esteem and mood in female subjects. What this means: "Low-intensity exercise may be just as good for the mind as it is for the body," says Dr. Rippe.

Q: **5. How can I prevent osteoporosis?**

A: We all build bone until about age 35, after which we lose 1 to 8 percent of our bone mass annually. Therefore, women should try to reach peak bone mass before age 35. This is especially important if osteoporosis runs in your family, putting you at an increased risk of developing the disease. The catch: "You can't achieve more than your genes will allow," says David Sartoris, M.D., director of the Bone Density Program at the University of California at San Diego School of Medicine.

Yet even though four-fifths of bone mass is determined by heredity, the remaining fifth that results from lifestyle choices can be important in preventing the disease. In fact, if you're below your peak, you may continue to gain bone into your late thirties and forties.

Calcium intake is crucial because "every organ in the body needs it," says Ethel Siris, M.D., professor of clinical medicine at Columbia—Presbyterian Medical Center in New York City. "If you don't take in enough calcium, your body will borrow it from your skeleton." Although adult women should consume 1,000 milligrams a day—the equivalent of four glasses of skim milk—half of us are getting less than 500. If your intake falls below the recommended level, make up the difference with a supplement or a digestive aid like Tums; it delivers 200 milligrams of calcium per tablet.

Exercise is also important to keep your skeleton healthy. Upper-body weight lifting and weight-bearing activities such as walking, jogging or biking at high resistance help you build bone mass in your twenties and maintain it later on.

A variety of lifestyle factors can also contribute to premature bone loss: frequent dieting, anorexia or bulimia, amenorrhea (common in some athletes), smoking and excessive alcohol intake. Certain medications may also leach bone from your body, including some prescribed for asthma, thyroid conditions and seizures.

Women with a family history of osteoporosis should have a bone-density test of the hip and spine taken about the time of menopause. Those who have had conditions or indulged in behaviors that put them at risk for the disease should be tested in their thirties. This painless x-ray, which is covered by some but not all private insurers, will tell you if your bone mass is above or below average for your age and help you and your doctor decide what course of action to take.

Q: 6. How can I assure myself the best prenatal care?

A: Doctors believe that to head off potential complications, prenatal care should begin prior to conception. For instance, if you haven't had German measles—which can cause serious birth defects if acquired during pregnancy—you should be immunized before becoming pregnant. If you have diabetes, which can lead to birth defects, a complicated delivery and a high-birth-weight baby, your blood sugar levels should be under control before you conceive, says Jennifer Niebyl, M.D., head of obstetrics and gynecology at the University of Iowa, Iowa City.

High blood pressure should also be controlled, as it can worsen during pregnancy, and STDs should be treated prior to, or at the very least during, pregnancy. Both conditions can cause premature delivery, according to Thomas Moore, M.D., director of perinatal medicine at the University of California at San Diego Medical Center.

In addition, early testing for genetic disorders such as Tay-Sachs disease, sickle-cell anemia and thalassemia will allow you time for risk counseling should the results be positive. Research has also recently underscored the value of getting at least 0.4 milligrams of folate (from green vegetables like broccoli and spinach, whole grains and citrus fruits) every day to prevent neural tube defects, which generally develop within 28 days of conception—before most women know they're pregnant.

Once pregnant, a woman should get regular checkups and may want to consider the following care.

Monitoring for multiple births. Due to the increased use of fertility drugs, the incidence of multiple births is rising dramatically, putting women at a greater risk of premature delivery. An electronic stethoscope-like instrument can usually detect the presence of extra heartbeats, and ultrasound can confirm the diagnosis.

Early ultrasound. While the American College of Obstetricians and Gynecologists does not recommend routine ultrasounds for all women, they are often performed at 18 to 20 weeks to confirm a due date and help detect fetal abnormalities. Regarding the safety of the procedure, Dr. Moore says that animal studies have shown that high levels of ultrasound early in pregnancy may reduce litter numbers and the growth of pups, but human studies have not shown negative effects.

Alpha-fetoprotein (AFP) test. Performed at 15 to 18 weeks, this new blood test reveals whether a woman may be at risk of delivering a baby with Down's syndrome. AFP, however, does not confirm a chromosomal defect. For that, a woman with a positive test would have to undergo amniocentesis.

Finally, Dr. Moore suggests finding out the following about any hospital you're considering using.

"Will I be allowed to get up and move around during labor?"

"Is epidural anesthesia available for pain control?" (Any hospital that uses an epidural in less than 10 percent of deliveries probably does not have it readily available, according to Dr. Moore.)

"What percentage of deliveries are performed by cesarean section?" The national average is 24 percent, but some hospitals have even higher rates. Hospitals are required to calculate their rates annually, so a figure should be available.

"If my baby has a difficult start at birth, who will be called in to help?" A pediatrician or nurse practitioner and respiratory therapist should be available around the clock, preferably in-house.

"How long may I have to bond with my baby right after birth?" Postdelivery, many hospitals take infants to a check-point for one to four hours to measure their vital signs. Ask in advance if the pediatric staff can conduct the physical exam while you're holding your baby in your arms.

Q: **7. What's the single most effective lifestyle change I can make for my health?**

A: If you smoke, stop. And whenever possible, avoid sec-ondhand smoke. Lung cancer is the number one cause of cancer death in women. It's estimated that 56,000 women will die of the disease this year, compared with 46,000 from breast cancer. The American Cancer Society estimates that more than three-quarters of these deaths will be a result of smoking—and therefore are preventable. "Women smoking cigarettes will come up to me at parties, worrying about breast cancer," says Bonnie Glisson, M.D., associate profes-sor of medicine at the University of Texas M. D. Anderson Cancer Center in Houston. "They have no idea they should be just as concerned about lung cancer."

While smoking has declined in women—from 33.9 per-cent in 1965 to 22.8 percent in 1990—women are at greater risk of dying from a smoking-related illness today than 30 years ago. That's because they are more likely to have begun smoking at an earlier age, to smoke more cigarettes per day and to inhale more deeply. In addition, by the year 2000, the prevalence of smoking is expected to be higher among adult women than it is among adult men because women are not quitting as fast as men are.

Lung cancer is especially dangerous because there are no gold-standard tests for early diagnosis. As a result, some 39 percent of cases are not detected until the disease has spread to distant organs. Currently, the five-year survival rate for these cases is only 2 percent.

It's never too late to kick the habit. A 1990 surgeon general's report showed that people who quit, regardless of age, live longer than those who continue to smoke.

Q: **8. With skin cancer on the rise, how can I avoid it?**

A: Americans have a 16 percent risk of developing basal cell and squamous cell cancers sometime during their lives, compared with a lifetime risk of less than 1 percent for malignant melanoma, the deadliest of skin cancers. But while melanoma is less prevalent overall, it is, according to the American Cancer Society, the most frequent cancer in women between the ages of 25 and 29 and the third most common (after breast and cervical cancer) in women aged 30 to 34.

Because people whose melanomas are caught early are almost always cured, doctors are encouraging us to examine our skin every three months. Use a hand-held and full-length mirror so you can see the front as well as the back of your body, and be on the lookout for a birthmark, mole or brown spot that has changed in color, size or texture; has an irregular outline; is bigger than a pencil eraser; or continues to itch, scab or bleed. Another tip: As it grows, melanoma frequently becomes raised and turns bluish-black in color.

"Self-examination has not been talked about enough," says Perry Robins, M.D., president of the Skin Cancer Foundation. "Yet there's no question that an increase in size of ¼ inch with a malignant melanoma can mean the difference between life and death." For any skin cancer, early detection may mean the difference between a simple excision and disfiguring surgery.

Promising advances are being made in the areas of prevention and treatment. According to Ronald Moy, M.D., co-chief of dermatology at the University of California at Los Angeles School of Medicine, one successful method of preventing precancerous lesions known as actinic keratoses from developing into skin cancer is to remove them with a light chemical peel. And researchers at the University of Arizona Health Sciences Center in Tucson and elsewhere are studying the effect of interferon injections on certain skin cancers. So far, the cure rate is 85 percent for basal cell and squamous cell carcinomas, says Kevin L. Welch, M.D., assistant professor of dermatology at the center.

Still, it pays to be vigilant about skin cancer prevention. The message doctors are imparting hasn't changed: Stay out of the sun between 10 A.M. and 3 P.M., the hours when ultraviolet (UV) rays are strongest, wear a hat with a wide brim on sunny days and daily use a sunscreen that blocks both UVA and UVB rays and has a sun protection factor (SPF) of at least 15.

Q: 9. Am I obeying the basic safety rules for avoiding accidents?

A: Injuries—in particular those resulting from motor vehicle accidents—are the leading cause of death among women under age 35. "The majority of women drivers killed in single-vehicle nighttime crashes have illegally high blood alcohol levels," says Susan Baker, professor of health policy and management at the Johns Hopkins School of Public Health in Baltimore and senior author of *The Injury Fact Book.*

Besides the obvious advice about not drinking and driving (the no-drinking rule applies to water sports such as boating and swimming as well), Baker urges women to always wear seat belts and to buy airbag-equipped cars.

When biking, wear a helmet and keep the chin strap fastened. "It's important to wear your helmet even if you're not riding in traffic," says Baker. Your head will be protected should you fall off your bike or hit a tree.

Don't overlook the risk of a household fire, another leading cause of accidental death among women. Make sure your home has a smoke detector with working batteries. If you're a homeowner, consider having a sprinkler system installed, says Baker.

Taking precautions during recreational activities is just as important. While sports injuries are rarely fatal, they can result in serious bone breaks and muscle and ligament strains. Most problems arise due to suddenly changing the intensity, duration or frequency of exercise. Abruptly increasing the duration, for instance, can result in an overuse injury like tendinitis. "A safe rule of thumb is to increase only one factor at a time, and by no more than 10 to 15 percent a week," says Robert Cantu, M.D., president of the American College of Sports Medicine.

Don't take up a new sport that uses completely different muscle groups without first conditioning regularly for several months. Going abruptly from an upper-body activity like rowing to downhill skiing is asking for trouble, says Dr. Cantu.

If you do experience a muscle pull or connective tissue sprain or strain, immediately stop the activity that caused it, apply ice for 20 minutes, compress the area with a supportive elastic bandage and elevate the affected limb. "If you do this right away, you'll help prevent swelling," says Peter Bruno, M.D., of the Nicholas Institute of Sports Medicine and Athletic Trauma in New York City. "And you may reduce your risk of developing arthritis later in life."

Q: 10. How can I fight for more federal funding for women's health care?

A: As consumers of health care, women have long been neglected. A much-publicized report by the General Accounting Office in 1990 indicated that women were not being included in major medical studies, and subsequent reports have shown a gender bias in everything from the treatment of AIDS to heart disease. "Women need to become active if we're ever going to change our health-care system," says Cindy Pearson, program director for the National Women's Health Network.

Almost every area of women's health needs increased funding, including breast cancer, lung cancer, heart disease, menopause, AIDS, osteoporosis, reproductive health and contraception.

If you want to get involved, start by finding out the names of your representatives in Congress. Then call or write and ask for a list of all the congressional bills related to women's health. Encourage your senator or representative to support any bills regarding women's health that are of interest to you. If you're short on time, consider making a donation to a health-care advocacy group such as the National Breast Cancer Coalition (P.O. Box 66373, Washington DC 20035), the National Women's Health Network (1325 G Street, N.W., Washington DC 20005) or the National Black Women's Health Project (1237 Ralph David Abernathy Blvd. S.W., Atlanta GA 30310).

—*Leslie Laurence*

PART TWO

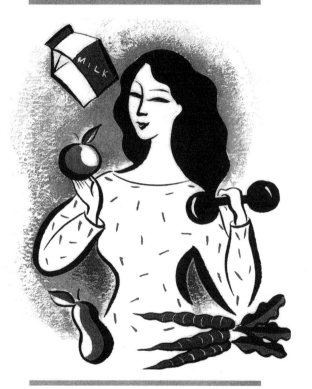

HOW TO EAT WELL
AND STAY TRIM

WHY IT'S SO TOUGH
TO LOSE THOSE
LAST TEN POUNDS

YOU'VE ALMOST WON THE WAR AND TAKEN OFF
THAT WEIGHT. HERE'S WHY THE FINAL BATTLE
IS THE MOST DIFFICULT.

If over time you've arrived at the sad conclusion that losing ten pounds and keeping them off is a lot harder than it sounds, you're right. As anxious as you are to reach your desired weight and stay there, you may have already discovered that this can be an exercise in futility.

Starting a diet is seldom a problem for most people, and the initial weight loss—a combination of water, protein, glycogen (blood sugar stored in the muscles and liver) and some fat—is always gratifying to see. But reaching your goal ultimately means losing body fat, and fat, unfortunately, is precisely what we gain when we gain weight and is the last thing to go when we lose weight. And when weight loss doesn't occur with the speed and ease we'd all like it to, many impatient dieters are apt to give up.

Yet the situation is far from hopeless. Understanding the physiological reasons for your last-ten-pounds diet woes will help you get past many of the hurdles if you do decide to diet—for the very last time.

BATTLING YOUR BODY

Your body is carefully and miraculously designed to keep you healthy and protect you from starvation—and it perceives dieting as gradual starvation. After all, when you diet you are deliberately withholding the body's usual supply of nutrients and energy sources. The body then starts to fight off this potentially dangerous depletion of energy stores by slowing down—and you may experience this as a weight-loss slowdown or even a plateau. The closer you are to your ideal weight and the less fat you have to lose, the more your body is going to cling tenaciously to what's already there.

Some experts label this the "set point," the weight at which your body struggles to remain, regardless of the outside pressures on it to change. "It's a push/pull phenomenon," explains nutritionist Judy Marshel. "When you diet, your body is fighting to release the fat, while at the same time your fat cells are constantly striving to fill themselves up with more fat."

SAY NO TO THE YO-YO

The "yo-yo" dieting syndrome further complicates things. Whenever you lose weight, you lose fat and some lean muscle mass; whenever you regain weight, you add only fat. So every time you put weight back on, you're changing your body's fat/lean muscle ratio—for the worse. With every subsequent attempt to lose weight, your body must struggle with more fat than it had the last time around. Then, when you don't see the weight come off despite all your genuine efforts, frustration usually—and understandably—sets in. Your what's-the-use? attitude may then lead to overeating and a regain of the lost pounds. Thus the loss/gain/loss/gain cycle begins once more.

Yo-yo dieting—or weight cycling, as it's currently called—can be more than just frustrating. Recent research shows it's also potentially dangerous to health. Kelly D. Brownell, M.D., a psychologist and weight specialist at Yale University in New Haven, Connecticut, published the results of a 32-year study of weight fluctuation in the *New England Journal of Medicine*. The risk of heart disease, including death from heart disease, was 25 to 93 percent higher in the group exhibiting the greatest amount of yo-yo dieting, regardless of how much or how little they weighed at the start. The study also revealed the added health risks to young females—the group most likely to be dieting in the first place—caused by yo-yo dieting. "The pressure in this society to be thin at all costs may be exacting a serious toll," Dr. Brownell concluded.

While his study is considered controversial and is not universally sanctioned within the professional nutrition and weight-loss community, most experts agree that weight cycling isn't good. Perhaps the biggest problem associated with it is the way it affects dieters psychologically. "It dates back to your very first diet," says Xavier Pi-Sunyer, M.D., director of endocrinology, diabetes and nutrition at St. Luke's–Roosevelt Hospital Center at Columbia University in New York City. "Most dieting problems are the psychological ones, the result of continuously trying and failing. That may be the biggest one you'll need to tackle."

CROSSING THE FINISH LINE

The ten-pounds-overweight dieter who has been losing/gaining/losing a small amount of weight for years has one type of problem. But the ten-pounds-overweight dieter who's successfully lost a lot of weight and is now nearing the diet finish line has a different dilemma. It has to do with the way the weight problem first began.

As a person gets heavier, the more fat accumulates in his fat cells, filling them up from the usual 0.5 microgram of fat per cell to their capacity of 1.0 microgram per cell. If the person gets heavier at that point, the existing fat cells will be unable to accommodate the excess, and so the body will start manufacturing more fat cells—extra cells you can never get rid of, no matter how hard you diet. What you'll accomplish if you do try to lose weight now will be to empty the fat out of the fat cells below their "normal" size, which your body will interpret as a signal that it's being undernourished. This situation makes you hungrier and drives you to eat more, so the body tends to "escape" from the diet it's on—and regain weight.

According to Dr. Pi-Sunyer, that's why very heavy dieters with these extra fat cells "have the hardest time of all returning to their normal weight—and it's probably unrealistic for them to even try." He believes such a person should forget about dropping the last ten pounds. "If someone went, say, from 150 to 300 pounds, she's better off trying to get down to about 175 than to her original 150."

BORN TO BE BIG

Another possible problem: You may be genetically predisposed to overweight. It's been shown repeatedly that if one of your parents is overweight, the likelihood of your being overweight increases by 40 percent. If both parents are overweight, your own chances are 80 percent greater. By inheriting your parent's extra number of (or larger-than-normal) fat cells, you become more vulnerable to a weight problem than someone with normal-weight parents.

Women dieters are also at a slight disadvantage compared with men. Women usually have more body fat than men, and that additional body fat means their bodies metabolize food less efficiently than men's.

Body size is another factor in weight loss. Because women tend to be physically smaller than men, women require fewer calories and a higher level of activity just to maintain their weight. Furthermore, if you're short and small-framed, you'll most likely need to consume fewer calories to lose or maintain your weight than your larger sisters and brothers.

EVER-SLOWING METABOLISM

Losing the last ten pounds is a challenge when you attempt to do it for the first time during middle age or later. That's because the older dieter generally must take in fewer calories than the younger dieter to accomplish a weight loss. Blame it on a slowing metabolism. Metabolic rate decreases by approximately 2 to 3 percent per decade, which means that your typical intake may now be adding pounds.

What's more, you may never have had even to think about dieting until recently. As a result, you might be having a tough time getting into the groove of counting calories and grams of fat and increasing your exercise. Change never comes easily, especially when you're older and when it involves something you've been doing all your life, such as eating.

You may also have a slight, chronic weight problem that's directly related to a particular medical condition and/or the medication you take for it. For example, cortico-steroids, used to treat rheumatoid arthritis, tend to cause water retention and stimulate the appetite. Clearly, as long as your condition persists, you're going to have an uphill battle trying to shed those last ten pounds. Consult with your doctor to see (1) if she believes dieting is even a good idea for someone with your condition, and (2) if she can recommend a strategy to help produce the desired weight loss.

You must also look at your few extra pounds within the context of your current lifestyle. For many people, eating and drinking—in restaurants, at the homes of friends and business associates, while traveling—are major social and business events. This is not to say that you can't control your intake in these situations; of course you can. However, it may be substantially more difficult for you than if you're someone who basically eats simply prepared meals at home. The struggle to maintain a ten-pounds-lower weight, when dining out is such an integral part of your work and leisure time, may honestly not be worth it.

DEALING WITH PLATEAUS

Usually at or close to the last-ten-pounds mark, many dieters hit a plateau. At that point it seems, no matter how diligent your dieting efforts, you can't get the needle on the scale to budge, for days or even weeks. "We don't know why it happens," admits Dr. Pi-Sunyer. "It might be fluid shifts, a redistribution of the sodium and potassium in the body or a variety of other reasons."

Naturally, it's frustrating when this occurs, but you know what you have to do: Stick to your diet and step up your activity level. If you become more energetic for a while, that will usually get you past the plateaus.

The weight-loss picture isn't nearly as bleak as this chapter may suggest. Any highly motivated dieter determined to see her weight loss to completion and beyond, regardless of her present circumstances, can do well. John Foreyt, Ph.D., director of the Nutrition Research Clinic at Houston's Baylor College of Medicine, insists that weight loss is within everyone's control. "People use genetics as an excuse for their weight, but the bottom line is lifestyle modification. My parents' genes don't determine how much I'm going to eat tonight or how much I'm going to exercise tomorrow—I do."

—*Linda Konner*

SIX SIMPLE RULES FOR EATING RIGHT

THESE EASY-TO-REMEMBER TENETS COVER ALL THE NUTRITION ESSENTIALS. THAT MEANS NO MORE AGONIZING OVER DETAILS—AND NO CALCULATOR REQUIRED.

More than a third of Americans think eating properly takes too much time, says a new report from the American Dietetic Association. And no wonder: With grams of fiber to be totaled, milligrams of calcium to be counted, percentages of fat and protein to be figured, you'd have to be a math whiz to achieve a balanced diet. "People are going nuts calculating this requirement and that," concedes Ruth Ann Carpenter, R.D., a nutritionist with the Cooper Institute for Aerobics Research in Dallas.

To make things easier, here are six easy-to-follow shortcuts based on interviews with leading nutritionists. Together these rules make it easy to maintain a healthy diet.

1. Abide by the great divide. Visualize your plate divided into quarters, then cover at least three-quarters with complex carbohydrates; foods from animal sources should occupy no more than a quarter of the plate. Experts tell us to emphasize grains, legumes, fruits and vegetables because they're low in calories and deliver plenty of health-enhancing fiber. Aim for as much variety as possible. For example, a plate piled with salad, wild rice and asparagus with a fillet of salmon is ideal for dinner.

2. Practice the palm principle. Eat a daily serving of protein that's about the size of your palm, says Sue Luke, R.D., a spokesperson for the American Dietetic Association. While many women worry that they don't get enough protein, most of them eat more than they need. A typical restaurant steak, for example, has 55 grams—that's up to 9 grams more than the daily requirement for women aged 19 and over. A palm-size piece of meat, poultry or fish is enough.

Legumes such as beans and peas are another excellent protein source, but be aware that these foods contain only half as much protein as animal foods.

3. Indulge once a day. Keep most of your meals lean, then feel free to have something sinful. Health mavens tell us to hold down fat in order to protect our hearts and reduce cancer risk. But you can afford a modest indulgence if you compensate by eating mostly low-fat foods, such as low-fat or nonfat dairy products, lean meats and low-fat baked goods. To avoid overindulging, steer clear of temptation by purchasing goodies by the serving.

4. Factor in five a day. Have at least five helpings of fruits and vegetables per day. Produce is not only high in fiber, it's rich in vitamins and minerals and will net you all you need, from vitamin A to zinc. Choose a variety of colors.

5. Do the daily double. Two servings of low-fat or nonfat dairy products will cover you on calcium. The evidence that calcium helps deter bone loss has made it a priority mineral for preventing osteoporosis. Now a study from the U.S. Department of Agriculture shows that eating the required amount may reduce the symptoms of premenstrual syndrome, too.

6. Shake a little. Choose fresh foods as often as possible, then sprinkle on a little salt if needed for taste. Even though the jury is still out about whether sodium raises blood pressure, most experts advise us to avoid high-salt fare. But the major culprits are processed foods, such as soups, canned vegetables and fast foods, not the salt shaker, according to a recent study. A few sprinkles on fresh food will add up to less sodium overall than you would get from a steady diet of processed foods.

—Daryn Eller

CAN THE FAT IMPOSTERS FAKE OUT YOUR TASTE BUDS?

AH, THE GREAT AMERICAN DREAM—THE TASTE OF FAT WITHOUT THE CALORIES. IT SOUNDS TOO GOOD TO BE TRUE . . . AND MAYBE IT IS.

As a nation addicted to chocolate and tortilla chips, we are not listening when nutritionists tell us that the best way to break the fat habit is to eat more whole grains, fruits and vegetables. Americans want what one expert calls a "techno-fix."

Ever eager to cater to Americans' couch-potato habits, the food industry is flexing its technological muscles to produce a range of processed foods with less or no fat. Considering that some 16 billion pounds of fat are added to processed food in this country every year, the market potential is enormous. But will fake fat revolutionize our diet?

Most of the engineered fats will be combined with other ingredients in processed foods. The new reduced-fat Milky Way II bar, for example, is made with Procter and Gamble's Caprenin, a reduced-calorie fat whose secret ingredient is behenic acid, a substance not easily metabolized by the body. Simple Pleasures, an ice cream substitute, and Kaukauna Cheese Lite 50 are made with Simplesse, a blend of microencapsulated whey proteins that mimic the "mouth feel" of fat.

Some salad dressings, puddings and frozen desserts use Oatrim, made from oat bran, which not only mimics the mouth feel of fat but also contains soluble fiber, which can help lower cholesterol. Since these fake fats are made from existing food components, they are not subject to rigorous Food and Drug Administration (FDA) testing.

GOOD FOR YOU?

In another category are entirely synthetic fats, such as Procter and Gamble's Olestra, a cooking oil replacement awaiting FDA approval. The agency considers these products "new food additives," which means they must be tested carefully before they're deemed fit for consumption.

But even if the new products are safe, it doesn't mean that their health value isn't questionable. It also remains to be seen if fat-reduced and fat-free products will help Americans eat a better diet, consume less fat and/or calories and control their weight.

Unfortunately, research shows that we have a complicated relationship with fat that tends to thwart such a simple solution. While it is not clear whether humans have an innate taste for fats (as we do for sweets), fat is a potent carrier of flavor, and most people, given the opportunity, eat a high-fat diet. Mimicking the mouth feel of fat may not be enough to satisfy that taste. Some provocative new studies even suggest that the proliferation of fat substitutes may actually encourage people to eat more high-fat foods.

So, given that we like what's bad for us, can we satisfy

FAT IN A FEW OF OUR FAVORITE THINGS

Food	Fat (g)
Piece of fruit	0–1.0
4 oz. flounder or sole	1–2.3
I cup cooked rice or pasta	0–2.0
Skinless chicken breast	4.0
I pat butter or margarine	4.0
I tsp. olive oil	4.7
I egg	6.0
I cup whole milk	8.0
¾ cup vanilla ice cream	10.5
Croissant	12.0
Avocado half	15.0
Slice of pecan pie	32.0
Double Whopper	53.0

our cravings and still keep our weight down? Not necessarily, says Robert Nicolosi, Ph.D., a clinical science professor at the University of Massachusetts at Lowell. "There isn't one bit of data that shows that eating a fat substitute or products enriched in fat substitutes helps maintain body weight," he says. "People just eat more calories."

Dr. Nicolosi concedes that the best way to lose weight is to cut fat, not just calories. One University of Illinois study showed that over five months, women who went on a diet with 20 percent calories from fat (down from 37 percent) lost weight, especially body fat, even when they ate more calories per day than they had previously. One reason is that our bodies can easily convert dietary fat into body fat, whereas we burn extra calories in the process of converting carbohydrates into body fat.

But, Dr. Nicolosi points out, low fat doesn't mean consequence free: If you eat a two-ounce piece of Entenmann's fat-free pound cake, there's no fat, but there are roughly 160 calories that have the potential to turn into body fat. If you eat an apple instead, again there's no fat, but there are only 65 calories. Obviously, you'll lose more weight eating apples than eating fat-free sweets.

WHAT ABOUT CALORIES?

One academic article written by scientists at Kraft General Foods estimates that if consumers substitute fat-free alternatives for such high-fat products as cheese, sour cream, salad dressings and baked goods, average daily fat intake would be reduced by about ten grams a day.

That's a significant savings for, say, a woman who consumes 1,800 calories a day and whose diet should include about 60 grams of fat, tops. But this assumes that we always substitute and don't cheat. Barbara J. Rolls, Ph.D., professor of biobehavioral health at Johns Hopkins University School of Medicine in Baltimore, is skeptical. She recently reviewed all the major scientific studies on the impact of low-fat foods on caloric intake and concluded that a supermarket full of fat-free and reduced-fat products may help people lower the percentage of fat in their diet, but it won't change the amount of calories they consume. Dr. Rolls's own research in the field supports this conclusion.

"In our studies, people make up the calories," she explains. In one such study Dr. Rolls gave healthy, normal-weight volunteers either a high-fat or low-fat lunch, without revealing which was which. They were free to eat whatever they wanted the rest of the day. On low-fat days, the subjects made up the calorie difference by dinnertime.

Another experiment, at Monell Chemical Senses Center in Philadelphia, revealed that people who thought they were on a low-fat diet but weren't ate more calories and more total fat. "It's the same story as saccharin with your coffee and a piece of pie," says Richard Mattes, R.D., Ph.D., who led the experiment with Florence Caputo, Ph.D. "You cheat a little more. If you use these products casually, they won't do anything for you."

An encouraging study conducted by Dr. Mattes suggests a better way to curb a high-fat appetite. In it, one group lowered its fat intake the usual way, by eliminating high-fat foods. After a month the members of this group began to prefer a lower level of fat in their diets. The other subjects were given fat substitutes. In this group, whose diet maintained the mouth feel of fat, there was no shift in fat preference.

"You can go on a low-fat diet, and eventually you'll come to prefer less fat in your diet—it's like salt," says Dr. Mattes. "Alternatively, you can rely on lower-fat products. Unfortunately, this blocks our built-in mechanism for adaptation."

In other words, either we can adjust to the pleasures of a naturally low-fat diet rich in breads, vegetables and fruits or, like methadone addicts, we can maintain our fat habit with substitutes.

—*Robert Barnett*

DIARY OF A DEMANDING DINER

BUTTER-LOVING COOKS, SNOOTY WAITERS AND MISLEADING MENUS—HOW'S A BODY SUPPOSED TO GET A HEALTHY MEAL?

Life could not have been easy for Mrs. Jack Sprat. Believe me, I know. The man with whom I hope to share all my tomorrows is on a strict low-fat, low-cholesterol, low-salt diet. Conversely, I am on a you-might-get-hit-by-a-truck-at-any-moment diet. I require dark Italian or Viennese roast with half-and-half; he drinks decaf with skim milk. I like my tuna folded into fluffy mayonnaise; he prefers his dry on a plate, like cat food. When he goes away, I fix myself three-cheese lasagna. When I'm out of town, he steams a whole mackerel. He insists all this vigilance will make him live longer. I tell him it will just seem that way.

BATTLING WELL-INTENTIONED WAITRESSES

Sometimes, when I don't want to strangle Howie, my heart fills with pity. The man's life is a quixotic crusade against the evil forces of sodium and butterfat. At times, even the culinary lexicon fails him. There was, I recall, the summer we spent traveling around Scotland, when Howie let his guard down—eating English breakfasts of porridge, scones, toast, eggs, sausage, ham and tomato. Finally forced to acknowledge a midsection no kilt could conceal, he steeled himself.

"Just one boiled egg," he instructed our hostess. "That's all." Minutes later, out she swooped, setting down a tray containing one egg—and toast, and a bowl of porridge, and sausage, and ham, and tomato. "I said *just one egg!*" Howie protested. "Oh, I *know* you did, love," our hostess chirped. "But we just didn't think one egg was enough breakfast for *any* soul, let alone a man of your size!"

Nor is the language problem any better closer to our home on Cape Cod. "I'd like a bagel, *no butter*," says Howie. The bagel appears under a golfball-size blob of cream cheese. "I'll take the grilled chicken sandwich, *just plain*," he offers patiently. The sandwich arrives minus lettuce and barbecue sauce, but the melted cheese, bacon and chicken fillet apparently are inseparable. In Maine, we found a waterfront restaurant that had "healthy heart" logos beside some entrées. Howie selected one; when it materialized it was barely visible under an avalanche of potato chips.

At home in our kitchen, where fat is banished, I have come to accept the virtues of steaming, poaching and grilling, of lemon juice, defatted chicken stock and nonfat yogurt. But dining out with Howie can be an ordeal. The scene is played out ad nauseam (and I mean nauseam): I select something from the menu, then try to make myself invisible while my mate does a *Five Easy Pieces* routine, verbally deconstructing an elaborate menu offering until he has, by default, ordered himself an ungarnished chicken breast.

According to the National Restaurant Association, Howie and I reflect a clear division among the restaurant-going public. There are three major categories of customers, says the association, which monitors prandial behavior with a zeal equal to that of Howie watching his cholesterol. "Committed patrons"—39 percent of the population, including Howie—exhibit dining behavior "consistent with their commitment to good nutrition." Then there are the "unconcerned patrons." Accounting for 32 percent of the population, they're the diners who don't bug the waitress, at least not about saturated fat. The rest fall into the category of "vacillating patrons," who care about their health but are "taste driven" when eating out. That would be me. I am taste driven and utterly unashamed of it. Who goes to Nathan's merely to stay alive?

ASSERTING YOUR LOW-FAT RIGHTS

Recently, though, I've found myself driven by motivations other than taste—in particular, by a pair of jeans that were obviously planted in my dresser drawer as a cruel joke. It was while fighting the zipper that I decided that perhaps I could afford to be more of a committed patron myself. After all, if I can happily devour nonfat meals at home, why shouldn't I at least go easy on the fat when eating out?

But I didn't look forward to crossing the line from perfect, passive customer to self-obsessed—I mean resolved and assertive—patron. Would I be ridiculed at busy chain restaurants? Would I be iced out of more exclusive ones? Would I have to resign myself to that dreaded dry breast of chicken at the tastiest of dinner spots? In her waitressing days, my friend Janet, pushed beyond the breaking point by a demanding customer, dumped the woman's entire meal in her lap. Was this the type of retribution I was in for?

I forced myself to think of those petite jeans when my friend Sara and I stopped in for dinner at Chili's, a restaurant specializing in the pan-fried, the deep-fried and the refried.

The waitress eyed us with something like disbelief as I asked whether the tostada chips were baked or fried. They were, of course, fried.

"Does the black bean soup have any sour cream in it?" I asked. "Or any fat?"

"No, it's just, you know, *from beans*," our waitress said with a roll of her eyes.

"Does it come with anything on it?" I heard Sara giggle. She sounded like I used to when I worried that Howie would take his questioning too far. When you're a size two like Sara, you can afford to laugh.

"Oh yeah, there's scallions . . . and cheese," the waitress said.

Sara and I decided on chicken fajitas for two, after the waitress told us the chicken was grilled and the onions sautéed in vegetable oil. I ordered soup—no cheese—and Sara, spotting "fresh steamed vegetables," asked for them dry.

The waitress took all this down. I mention it only because the vegetables arrived under an unmistakable slick of butter, and the "just beans" in my black bean soup seemed to have sprouted hunks of salty smoked sausage. We didn't eat much. "I'm not going to offer *you* two dessert," the waitress said with a smirk as she handed us the check.

I paid without a word.

Which, I suppose, is not what is meant when the American Heart Association counsels diners to be assertive. "Remember that you are the patron," advises the association's *Guide to Restaurant Dining.* "Ask questions. Don't be intimidated by the menu, the atmosphere, your waiter or waitress . . . . Insist that food be served the way you want it."

BLESS THE SAVVY RESTAURATEURS

Clearly, it was time to let a pro take over. The next time out, Howie and I headed for Gruber's, a cozy bistro tucked into an alley off Provincetown's main street. As we perused the list of appetizers, my head rang with echoes of *Wayne's*

World: Caesar salad . . . *not!* Fried crab cakes . . . *not!* I felt a pang of empathy for Howie, who goes through this all the time. Wait, here's asparagus with smoked salmon . . . and red pepper hollandaise.

Howie began his cross-examination as I tried not to cringe. "The pan-fried sole . . . is that fried in butter or oil? Could I get it without the citron butter?"

Our waitress was unfazed. "We could fry it in vegetable oil for you," she said.

Howie followed up, "Is the grilled tuna cooked with butter? Is it seasoned with salt? The pasta, is that prepared with any butter or cream? Are your vegetables steamed or sautéed? Sautéed in what?"

It was one of Howie's best performances. Yet our waitress obliged us so solicitously, her brow furrowed in concern, that one would have thought that what was being sold here was real estate, not ephemeral food. I don't know how she maligned us once she hit the kitchen, but her tableside manner was nothing short of maternal, "Are you all right here? Is everything okay?" Even, bless the woman, *"Do you have any more questions?"*

Maybe she wasn't making faces behind the kitchen door at that. According to the restaurant association, seven out of ten adults restrict their fat intake, which means that ignoring nutritional concerns has become as bad for a restaurant's business as it is for the patron's health. Says Michael Horowitz, waiter at Ciro and Sal's in Provincetown, diners worry unnecessarily about special requests. "Nothing you can ask for will surprise us," says Horowitz. "We've heard it all before."

HELP MAY BE NEAR

Good waiters and waitresses see themselves as the diner's emissary to the kitchen, Horowitz says. They often know as much as the chef about the dishes they serve, so listen carefully to the dramatic reading of the menu: Especially in upscale places, *nothing* is left to the imagination.

"Hi, I'm Kevin," says your waiter. "This evening we're serving Sri Lankan duck that has been dried, pummeled, driven to the Canadian border and back, then tossed in a shallot burgundy butter with a champagne bing cherry glaze and served on a bed of *chèvre*-stuffed shiitake ravioli." After such a soliloquy, you may wish Kevin would get on with his acting career—but you'll also have the information you need to make healthful choices.

Still, I worried about resistance at high-toned restaurants that specialize in the butter-based sauces whose laborious preparation dominates much of prime-time public television. At Chillingsworth, an exceedingly elegant, extraordinarily pricey French country restaurant in Brewster, Massachusetts, Howie and I sat in the hush of a Victorian drawing room puzzling over "sweet pepper mousse," "garlic custard," "lobster cognac cream" and "lemon sorrel butter sauce." I was resigned to the prospect of lengthy negotiations before ordering, but shortly into our questions the waitress cut us short.

"Oh, I get it," she said. "You want something delicious but you're trying to be good." And she began to translate. Watch out for the hazelnuts on the brandied snails, she said, and stay away from the *dauphinois* potatoes—they're creamed. She offered to replace the butter sauce on the salmon with a light stock reduction and scrap the garlic custard for a basic vegetable, but we decided on tenderloins of beef and veal. They were so lean a cardiologist might have prescribed them, yet so tender you'd think they'd been drenched in butter. You couldn't get much further from the tasteless chicken breast of my nightmares.

For people who still love to eat for the sheer joy of it, the good news is that the increasing national vigilance regarding fat and salt has forced chefs to turn to more varied and subtle flavorings. Instead of piling on butter as a simple shortcut to taste, chefs are using fresh herbs and flavorful reductions—simmering down beef, chicken or vegetable stock into sauces for concentrated flavor.

And if you don't see what you want on the menu, you

can ask for modifications. "You don't even hear shrieking in the kitchen anymore," says Jody Adams, nationally known chef at Michela's, in Cambridge. Unless you ask for the impossible: Cooks can take the egg out of the Caesar salad, but they can't take the cheese out of fettuccine Alfredo. There's no such thing as meuniére or béarnaise sauce without the butter, or hollandaise without the eggs.

On the other hand, a chef *can* make a lovely marsala sauce without a bit of butter. Though fish can't be grilled without oil—it would stick to the grill—it can be broiled that way. So can chicken. Let your waiter know what you're after, says Gianfranco Verri, a waiter at Boston's exclusive Ritz-Carlton; the chef may be able to come up with a tasty solution. "People automatically ask about the fat in our sauces," says Verri. "Often, we can use a light, simple sauce of olive oil and white wine or the natural juices of the meat. Our chef takes a lot of pride in his work. He won't serve plain, bland food."

IT PAYS TO ASK

Special requests make sense in an elegant restaurant. After all, I'm signing over most of my paycheck in return. But when Howie and I wanted to grab a meal before a movie, I wasn't sure whether a family-style chain restaurant would be willing to lean over backward to please a picky eater.

At Lum's, though, no leaning was required. Nearly 90 percent of chain restaurants have switched to vegetable oil for frying, according to the National Restaurant Association. Most list some variety of light fare and offer broiled or grilled entrées. And all the offerings are in plain English. Instead of puzzling over scallop glazes, Howie and I mulled over spaghetti sauce. We didn't ponder coq au vin; we considered chicken sandwiches. We got our baked potatoes dry and our fish and chicken grilled and butter free. And when Howie asked for coffee, he was able to get skim milk for it. My finicky mate was thrilled. Most restaurants don't stock anything below 2 percent.

But Lum's offers its dinner patrons unlimited visits to its salad bar. Who could imagine such wickedness? At least 15 of the 60 or so offerings were drowned in mayonnaise, not to mention the creamy dressings and oil-soaked croutons. When my chaste chicken fillet arrived, I was too stuffed to eat more than a bite or two.

I guess I missed a phase in my metamorphosis into healthy diner. When I was growing up, eating out always meant an hour of obscene overindulgence followed by a car ride throughout which my family gasped like a school of

THE WAITER SUGGESTS

Gianfranco Verri has served dinner at Boston's Ritz-Carlton for 20 years. Michael Horowitz has been a waiter for the past 11 years and works at Ciro and Sal's, a bustling Provincetown trattoria that serves as many as 350 meals on a typical Saturday. I asked them to offer advice on how we can make life easier on ourselves when we dine out.

• If you have special dietary needs, it's best to fess up immediately. If before ordering you say, "I'm watching my fat intake," or "My doctor has me on a low-salt diet," the waiter can make special menu suggestions or consult the chef.

• With their power to create delicious dishes, chefs in good restaurants are reluctant to serve bland food. "People have asked for just a plain veal cutlet instead of veal parmesan," says Horowitz. "The chef can do that very easily, of course, but it offends his sensibility. He doesn't want unappetizing meals served in his restaurant." Let your server know what you're after, but be willing to leave the details to the chef, Horowitz suggests. Many take a low-fat request as a challenge to their creativity.

• Listen to your waiter or waitress. "We've had customers insist we serve them something like beached whales, our clothing unzipped. In years past I lived a simple truth: The more delicious a meal, the more profound the agony that follows it. And yet, it occurred to me, I'd never begin a meal at home by eating four buttered slices of bread or a triple helping of salad.

All the hoopla over fat and cholesterol in recent years seems to be obscuring a crucial point: When we eat out, we eat too much. Many chefs, Julia Child among them, insist that there are no "bad foods." The key to a healthy diet is variety and moderation. When the people at the American

nondairy pesto," says Horowitz. "We just can't do that—the pesto's already been prepared. But I can direct any diner to 20 nondairy, nonfat dishes on our menu."

• Arm yourself with a little knowledge about the cuisine you favor, Verri suggests. Education comes with dining experience, of course. But many cookbooks have eminently readable sections profiling the character of a particular cuisine, and restaurant reviews can also offer a guide. Savvy diners know an Italian kitchen can produce a special order of pasta dressed with garlic and olive oil, for instance. And even if it's not on the menu, fish broiled without butter is always available at a French restaurant.

• Don't be shy about grilling your waiter—after all, it's better than being shocked when the food arrives. Horowitz and Verri both say they'd rather deal with a lot of questions than with a dissatified customer.

• Remember that for each special request, your waiter must make an earnest plea to the harried chef. "On a busy night," says Horowitz, "we waiters get our heads chopped off." Some waiters don't feel it's worth the effort. You can make it so by leaving a generous tip of 20 percent or more.

Heart Association tell you that no more than 30 percent of your calories should come from fat, they're referring to your *overall* diet.

You needn't banish the creamy, the crispy and the buttery, as long as you eat less of it. Have a little of your entrée and take the rest home. Or order an appetizer-size portion of your favorite dish and share the dessert. And if you're going out for a once-a-year fling, budget your calories, fat and cholesterol in the days before and after, so you can be carefree at the restaurant table.

THREADING THE ETHNIC MAZE

Once-a-year flings are not an option for me. I find it absolutely necessary to visit an Indian restaurant at least once a month. My friend Pat, equally enamored of the cuisine, usually comes with me. So she was horrified when I told her, on our way to our local favorite, that I planned to hold to my low-fat regimen. If we alienated the good people at Pavilion Indian Cuisine, Pat pointed out, our next curry would require a 2½-hour drive to Boston.

But I was convinced that ethnic food would be an ideal choice for the new, Howie-esque me, a way of going heavy on the flavor without much fat. I knew I'd face changes as I ate my way around the world. Calvin Trillin once wrote that the only thing he wants to learn to say in Chinese is "I'll have what they're having," but if you aim to avoid coconut milk in Thai cooking, cottonseed oil in Chinese cuisine or fried food the world over, you have to climb the language barrier.

Luckily, I'd been eating Indian food long enough to know that I should ask the cook to substitute vegetable oil for ghee—butter that's been clarified but is just as bad for you as the cube variety. But until the waiter warned me, I was unaware of the cream concealed in *baingan bhartha*, my favorite dish of spicy mashed eggplant. Ignorance is bliss, I thought regretfully, until he continued, "I will make sure the cook leaves the cream out."

He positively enthused as he placed the steaming platters before us. "No butter or cream in any of it!" Much of the flavor of Indian food comes from spices, sweet burned onions and yogurt-based sauces. I would have told our waiter that I didn't miss the fat at all—not in the eggplant, the chicken simmered with spinach or the spicy okra dish—but my mouth was full.

I was feeling pretty cocky when I grabbed Howie a week later and headed for Boston's Chinatown. In the short time I'd been a committed diner, I'd tamed my fear of snooty waiters and fearlessly asked for menu alterations in the haughtiest halls of haute cuisine. Now I'd even found the ethnic shortcut to healthy, tasty restaurant dining.

At the Lucky Dragon, our waiter endured our interrogation with only an occasional roll of the eyes. He was a gentle, patient soul—also, we appeared to be the only customers in the place.

Considering our pickiness, the most aptly named selection on the menu was U-toy with oyster sauce, but that was on the forbidden list, and nothing around here was being grilled except our hapless waiter. So we went with steamed dumplings and steamed chicken with black mushrooms, to avoid the oil that drenches so many Chinese dishes. We also ordered *moo shi* chicken and shrimp with black bean sauce. But hold the MSG and the salt, I said, and give us the soy on the side. The waiter now glanced at us with something like pity. "I can do it," he said somberly. "But I must tell you, no MSG, no salt, no soy . . . no taste!"

When the dishes arrived, they looked well, peculiar. In fact, they looked exactly alike, which is to say colorless and nondescript. Why isn't the black bean sauce black? "No soy!" the waiter thundered.

Humbled, we filled our plates. Nothing had the faintest hint of a taste. For the first time in my life, I left a Chinese restaurant hungry. If I ate like this all the time, I mused, I'd probably live a lot longer. Or maybe it would just seem that way.

—*Susan V. Seligson*

SHORTCUTS
TO FITNESS

EVERYDAY ACTIVITIES—TALKING ON THE PHONE,
PLAYING WITH THE KIDS—CAN ADD UP.

You don't have a second to spare in your day for exercise. Although you have tried countless times, you've never been able to stick with a workout routine.

Your house is much too small to accommodate bulky exercise equipment. You can only dream of being able to afford one of those expensive health-club memberships. Besides, you'd be much too embarrassed to prance around in front of an aerobics class full of women—and men—who are thin, fit and gorgeous. So you're a hopeless case, right?

Wrong! You don't have to spend hours a week at a gym to get in shape. You can improve your health and fitness—and look and feel a lot better—by incorporating even small doses of physical activity into your day. As a matter of fact, you hardly even have to break a sweat!

Ridiculous, you say? Not at all, according to the most recent findings from the nation's leading exercise experts. "The fitness gurus used to insist that we had to punish ourselves with strenuous aerobic exercise for at least 30 minutes three times a week to get fit," says Bryant Stamford, Ph.D., director of the Health Promotion Center at the University of Louisville School of Medicine in Kentucky and author of *Fitness without Exercise.* "But new studies show major benefits from exercise so modest it doesn't feel like a workout."

A recent study involving 102 women between the ages of 20 and 40 at the Cooper Institute for Aerobics Research in Dallas showed that strolling a 20-minute mile—a lap or two around the typical mall—significantly decreases blood pressure and cholesterol levels, which reduces the risk of heart disease. "For lowering cholesterol and blood pressure, moderate exercise works as well as a strenuous workout," says John Duncan, Ph.D., associate director of the Cooper Institute and senior coauthor of the study. "And the more out of shape you are, the more you will benefit from doing low-intensity exercise."

Another study conducted at the University of Massachusetts Medical School in Worcester showed that even moderate walking reduces tension and anxiety. "No matter how slowly they walked, everyone felt less stressed afterward," says study author James M. Rippe, M.D., director of the university's Exercise Physiology and Nutrition Laboratory. In fact, these studies and others have helped convince the American Heart Association to promote modest exercise a few times a week as an excellent way to significantly reduce the risk of heart attack, currently the leading killer of American women.

"The health benefits of low-level exercise are great news for sedentary Americans," Dr. Duncan says. "Intensity doesn't matter. What is most important is regularity. If you become even slightly more active—and stick with it—your health will improve."

EXCUSES, EXCUSES

Everyone starts with the best of intentions. But all too often, we wind up making excuses for why we can't make time for fitness. Do any of these sound familiar?

"I'm just too busy." Of course you're busy. You lead a hectic life. That's more reason to exercise—to help manage your stress and build the self-esteem, stamina, strength and flexibility you need to cope with all the daily demands you face.

"I don't have large blocks of time to exercise." "You don't need them," Dr. Rippe says. "Sporadic exercise adds up. If you take just three 10-minute walks a day during breaks, you're exercising for 30 minutes."

What kind of physical activities do you already engage in? Shopping, cooking, child care? Stretch, bend and lift more during housework. Walk briskly while running errands. Get physical when you play with your children.

"I hate exercise." Don't sign up for water aerobics if you hate to swim. Choose a physical activity you like and do it regularly. You don't have to run, do sit-ups and use a stair-climbing machine. Even gardening or a nightly stroll burns calories.

"I've never been active. It's too late to start now." A recent study shows that even 90-year-old lifelong fitness-phobics gained significant physical and emotional benefits from modest, regular exercise. No matter how long you've been out of shape, it's never too late to get fit. Just start now and keep at it.

"I feel self-conscious. I'm a klutz when I exercise and I look terrible in tights." You don't look ridiculous. You look like a woman who's taking control of her life and health. You look great! Besides, everyone else is too busy obsessing about the way they look to worry about you.

"I never seem to improve." Be patient. It takes a month or two to notice the aerobic payoffs of exercise, and a while longer for any physical changes to appear. Keep a record of your progress. Make a chart that shows how many blocks from work you park or how many flights of stairs you can climb before you feel winded—anything that you can measure. Plot your progress on a weekly basis. Before you know it, you're sure to see some improvement.

"I can't afford to join a gym or turn my home into one." You don't have to. Do-it-yourself workouts—like housework and walking—don't cost a penny!

"I never stick with it." You're not alone. Half of those who start exercising give it up within 12 months.

To keep from being a quitter, follow these steps:

• Be realistic. For every year you've been out of shape, it takes a month to get fit again. What's more, remember that you may not reap the physical benefits exercise until six to eight weeks have passed. But you'll begin to feel the emotional benefits almost immediately.

- Start slowly and don't overdo it. You should be able to carry on a conversation while exercising. If you find yourself becoming breathless, you may be pushing too hard.
- Do only activities that feel fun. If one type of exercise isn't enjoyable, switch to another. Getting exercise shouldn't turn into a chore.
- Find a buddy. It's much easier to stick to a regular fitness routine when you exercise with a friend.
- Vary your activities. You'll be less likely to get bored and lose interest in working out.

FITNESS FIXES

There are plenty of simple shortcuts you can do to integrate more physical activity into your daily life. "Choose two or three and commit to doing them every day," recommends Ralph LaForge, director of health promotion at the San Diego Cardiac Center Medical Group.

Try walking up the stairs instead of taking the elevator. If you're out of shape, start by walking down the stairs. When climbing stairs no longer leaves you winded, climb a little faster.

Park a few blocks farther away. Walk the extra distance to work, the mall, the movies, church or friends' homes. As you gain stamina, park even farther away and walk more briskly.

Stash a pair of walking shoes at work. Slip them on for walks at lunch. Better yet, take a daily ten-minute stroll before lunch. You may discover that you'll want to eat less lunch afterward.

Buy a backpack. Then instead of driving around town when doing your errands, walk as much as possible and use the backpack to hold your purchases.

Avoid "food dates." Instead of meeting friends for lunch, coffee or dessert, make arrangements to take walks, go dancing or shopping, visit a museum or go for bike rides together.

Walk your dog. If you don't have one, borrow a neighbor's. Dogs are great exercise companions.

Make breaks count. During television commercials or breaks at work, get up and stretch or walk around. Encourage co-workers and family members to join you. Use the opportunity to chat.

YOUR BEST EXERCISE INVESTMENT: GOOD SNEAKERS

Forget expensive health clubs, exercise equipment and designer sweats. You don't need them to get fit. But good sneakers are essential to even modest exercise programs.

• Check your feet. if you are flat-footed, you need extra arch support. If you have a high arch, you need extra shock absorption. For weak ankles, consider high-tops.

• Check your old sneakers. Notice where they're most worn and look for shoes reinforced in those areas.

• Shop in the afternoon. Feet swell during the day.

• Don't get overwhelmed by the different types of sneakers. Worry less about whether they're cross-trainers or aerobic sneakers and instead concentrate on the quality and features.

• Get the right fit. Experts say there should be about $\frac{1}{4}$ inch between your toes and the tip of the sneaker.

• Try on both sneakers. Feet vary greatly in size.

• Check the weight. The lighter the better.

• Check the traction. Shoes should not slip on any surface.

• Test them. Sneakers should feel comfortable in the store. They shouldn't require breaking in. Jump up and land on your forefeet. In well-cushioned shoes, you should feel almost nothing. Rock from side to side. You shouldn't wobble. Pivot in different directions. Your shoes should always feel flexible.

Don't automatically use the phone or intercom at work. Walk to your co-workers' desks instead.

Make the most of phone time. Don't sit while talking—pace instead. Invest in a longer handset cord so you can walk farther, or get a cordless phone.

If you must stand in one spot, march in place, raising your knees up high. Or rise up on your tiptoes. Do this five times, then do five half-knee bends. Gradually work up to doing ten repetitions.

Another telephone tip: Keep a small three-pound weight or a can of food near the phone and, while talking, do weight-training curls and presses.

Curls: With your arm straight, hold the can or weight down by your hip. Bend your elbow and bring the weight up to your shoulder.

Presses: Start with your arm in the curled position, then straighten it over your head. Do five of each. When you feel ready, do ten.

Make the most of "microwave minutes." Don't stand around thinking about the snack you're going to scarf down. Pace, stretch or do some calisthenics.

Put more energy into housework. Scrubbing floors, vigorously sweeping and vacuuming, washing the windows and other chores provide more exercise than you might think. What's more, if you step up the pace you will finish much sooner—and get a worthwhile workout as well.

Make the most of time spent unpacking groceries. Curl and press cans a few times. When you feel ready, try it with six-packs.

Don't always automatically reach for the food processor. When time permits, cut, chop and dice all those vegetables by hand.

Wash and iron your own clothes. You'll get a workout and save on laundering. Spend that money on something exercise-related, such as a dancing class or an aerobics tape.

Work outdoors. Pushing a power mower is great aerobic exercise. Or retire your power mower and invest in a push model. Digging, weeding, raking and shoveling are also good—for the body and the mind.

Here are a few more tips just for mothers:

Walk your baby. Infants love motion. Put your baby in a backpack or carriage and take a stroll to the park or the store.

Weight-train with your baby. Play with your little one on the floor. Lift her overhead, exercise her arms and legs.

Push your child. Kids love swings and merry-go-rounds. Pushing them provides you with great exercise.

Join in older children's games. Play tag. Go roller skating. Jump rope. Climb a play structure. Take a swim, a bike ride or a rowboat outing on a lake. You'll have so much fun that you might not even notice that you're exercising.

—*Michael Castleman*

I'D KILL FOR A COOKIE

WHEN THOSE ABSOLUTELY-HAVE-TO-HAVE-IT FOOD URGES REACH OUT AND GRAB YOU, WHY IS IT THAT YOU NEVER, EVER FANTASIZE ABOUT BROCCOLI? FIND OUT HOW TO CONQUER INSIDIOUS FOOD CRAVINGS.

For Sarah, it's a chocolate fit every month just before she gets her period. After a tough day at the office, Nancy covets tortilla chips. Debbie suddenly can't resist cheese—one reason she's slowly regaining the 40 pounds she just lost.

Most of us have experienced a strong, nearly uncontrollable urge for a certain type of food. And while we've struggled to keep ourselves from the refrigerator, we may have wondered why we long so intensely for one food. Here is what researchers are learning about cravings—why they start, what they mean and how to control them.

BORN TO CRAVE

Yearnings are as individual as yearners themselves, but nearly all are for foods high in sugar, salt or fat. Think about it: When's the last time you would have sold your soul for a stalk of celery?

"People just don't crave vegetables or a slice of whole-grain bread," says Audrey T. Cross, Ph.D., professor of nutrition at the Columbia School of Public Health in New York City. In fact, she says, this has been proven: When a group of subjects were shown pictures of chocolate cake, they salivated; pictures of broccoli had no effect.

But our cravings may not be as depraved as they seem: They start out as healthy needs in childhood. Breast milk is sweet and salty, so it makes sense that we're born liking these tastes. With sodium, too, we may be fulfilling a need for this vital nutrient that controls the movement of fluid in and out of cells. "Most animals will instinctively seek out salt when they're depleted," says Judith S. Stern, Sc.D., professor of nutrition and internal medicine at the University of California, Davis. Animals look for salt licks, while people will choose a snack of pickles, potato chips or pizza with anchovies.

As for yearnings for high-fat foods, these foods are necessary in the very early years to sustain rapid growth. But even when children outgrow their biological needs, their tastes persist, as passions turn to peanut butter and jelly, cheeseburgers and milk shakes, and for the more sophisticated palate of adults, Rocky Road ice cream and creamy chocolate mousse.

WHAT DO WOMEN REALLY WANT?

Raiding the refrigerator is not a gender-linked activity, but cravings are more common in women. And though both men and women seek fatty foods, we like ours packaged with high-sugar carbohydrates—such as candy, cake and cookies. Men usually want foods that are high-protein, high-fat combinations, like steak and french fries, cheeseburgers, sausage or hot dogs, says Adam Drewnowski, Ph.D., director of the Human Nutrition Program at the University of Michigan in Ann Arbor.

For years, researchers assumed these preferences were learned—that men simply thought it was more manly to choose meat over "wimpy" treats like whipped-cream cake. "But I was surprised to find that lab animals show the same preferences," says Dr. Drewnowski. Female rats select carbohydrate/fat mixtures, while male rats select protein/fat mixtures. This means, he says, that our choices may be physiological.

HEALTHY WAYS TO HANDLE CRAVINGS

In most instances, it's fine to indulge your food desires. But some of us do need to practice restraint: salt cravers who have high blood pressure; people who are overweight or have high cholesterol; and those who tend to binge if a craving is indulged. For these people or anyone who wants to gain more control of her eating habits, experts offer these strategies.

If you crave carbohydrates or sweets:

• Choose low-fat versions of the flavors you desire. Instead of sandwich cookies, choose plain graham crackers or animal crackers. Instead of ice cream, have low-fat frozen yogurt. Try satisfying the urge for milk chocolate with chocolate jelly beans or hard candies. Reach for a bagel with jam instead of a muffin with butter.

• Try eating a small amount of a low-fat, high-carbohydrate food before a meal. Otherwise you may stuff yourself in a futile attempt to feel satisfied but then go ahead and eat dessert anyway, since what you really wanted was the carbohydrate.

• If you begin a weight-loss program, be sure it includes a variety of textures, tastes and consistencies, including carbohydrates.

If you crave salt:

• Select low-fat substitutes: popcorn or pretzels

Menstrual cycles can set off specific urges. When we suffer premenstrual symptoms such as severe mood swings, our desire for sweet and starchy carbohydrates may surge, says Judith J. Wurtman, Ph.D., a research scientist in the Department of Brain and Cognitive Science at the Massachusetts Institute of Technology in Cambridge. But experiments show that a bowl of cornflakes can improve moods dramatically, "as if women had taken a Valium," says Dr. Wurtman.

The lift is provided by serotonin, a brain chemical that's

instead of potato chips, tortillas toasted under the broiler rather than packaged corn chips.

• If you need to avoid salt for a medical reason, experiment with various herbs and spices to stimulate your taste buds. And try salt-free versions of your favorite foods; you will get used to the taste.

If you reach for certain foods to relieve stress:

• When you crave crunchy, chewy foods, go for carrot and celery sticks, licorice, popcorn, sugarless gum or fruit.

• For smooth and creamy "comfort food" yearnings, try applesauce, nonfat cottage cheese and low-fat frozen yogurt.

To help resist temptation:

• Vary your travel routes so you don't walk or drive by the bakeries and ice cream stores that trip your trigger with their aromas or advertising.

• If you often crave the same food at the same time, break your routine. Instead of buying candy every afternoon when the coffee cart arrives, visit the rest room and brush your teeth or freshen your lipstick. Better yet, take a five-minute walk.

• Exercise regularly. Studies of lab animals show that active animals choose a diet lower in fat than animals that don't exercise.

produced after eating starches. It can cause those feelings of pleasure and satisfaction that people experience after a good meal. And since serotonin levels drop just before your period, your body will look for ways to pump them back up.

Also premenstrually, metabolic rates go up; our bodies are burning calories faster and want more fuel. If we eat more, it's likely that some fat will be stored—one way nature prepares the body for pregnancy in case of conception. We may also have a heightened sense of smell before our periods, which can exaggerate any food preferences.

The food premenstrual women crave most? Chocolate. No one knows why, but theories range from the obvious—that chocolate is high in fat and sugar and tastes good—to the more esoteric—that chocolate contains endorphins, chemicals that act as natural painkillers and antidepressants. In effect, premenstrual women may be "self-medicating" depression or mood swings by reaching for a chocolate bar.

Once our periods begin, many of us crave red meat. Is the body trying to replace the iron lost through monthly bleeding? Researchers say there's no evidence of this, although "it may be some conscious or subconscious nutrition knowledge at work," surmises Dr. Drewnowski.

As for the cliché about pregnant women lusting for pickles and ice cream, scientists have never proven that many actually do have the urge. (But it would almost make sense if they did: Ice cream is high in fat and sugar, reflecting the body's need for more calories. And pickles are high in salt, necessary because pregnancy increases the blood volume and eating salty foods can help women maintain the proper balance of sodium.)

Food preferences during pregnancy may also be caused by hormonal influences on the sense of taste, says Seattle dietitian Marilyn Guthrie, R.D., a spokesperson for the American Dietetic Association. In many pregnant women, this shows up in the form of food aversions—a strong dislike for dishes previously enjoyed. But except for salt, there's little evidence to suggest that a pregnant woman's cravings reflect her nutritional needs any more than anyone else's. Broccoli still isn't the object of desire.

Occasionally, some pregnant women want to eat non-food substances: baking soda, coffee grounds, cornstarch, even chalk or clay. These unnatural cravings, called pica, may indicate an iron deficiency. All cases of pica should be treated by a physician—the habit can prevent women from getting the nutrients they need.

HIGH ON FAT

Though nearly everyone experiences an occasional craving, some people have them intensely and often. They've been dubbed "carbohydrate cravers" by researchers, but many scientists now think the primary craving may be not for carbohydrates but for *fats.* "If people wanted pure carbohydrates, they'd eat plain bread or pasta or simple hard candies or sugar," says Allen Levine, Ph.D., deputy associate chief of staff for research at the Veterans Department of Affairs in Minneapolis. "Instead, people crave foods high in both sugar and fat, such as cookies, ice cream and chocolate candy."

Again, it may be chemicals—serotonin and endorphins—at work. Block the brain's ability to absorb these chemicals—as researchers have done in experiments with women who have intense food cravings (bulimic and overweight women)—and people are less likely to feel cravings or go on binges, reports Dr. Drewnowski.

These brain chemicals may be one reason some dieters have so much trouble maintaining their desired weight. After a certain period of time denying the cravings for fats and carbohydrates, the mind and body simply rebel. Some researchers believe that the whole phenomenon of yo-yo dieting—losing weight, then regaining it, then losing it again—is really a cycle of addiction and withdrawal and addiction again to the pleasurable brain chemicals that some foods produce.

People who don't have a weight problem may simply

not be as sensitive to these shifts. "Thin people experience food cravings, but not nearly as much as those who are overweight," says Susan Schittman, Ph.D., professor of medical psychology at Duke University in Durham, North Carolina. "When you ask overweight people for lists of what they crave, you get longer lists and a greater variety of flavors and textures—creamy, chewy, crunchy, crispy—than you get from others."

FOODS FOR STRESS RELIEF

Eating can also be an anxiety antidote. "While men tend to use exercise and other physical outlets, women may turn to food," says Guthrie.

For some, it's the chewing itself that relieves tension. Not surprisingly, the foods these stressed-out women tend to crave are crunchy—cookies and potato chips—or tough and chewy, like taffy or caramel-filled candy bars.

For others, soft, smooth, creamy foods—such as puddings, oatmeal and ice cream—are the most soothing. These so-called comfort foods may relieve stress because people associate them with pleasant feelings. "If your mother gave you tapioca whenever you were sick and then you felt better, tapioca can be a comforting food for you," explains Dr. Stern.

LEARNED LONGINGS

Other cravings are born of habit. Many of us became accustomed to highly salted foods in childhood, for example, and learned to prefer the taste. But interestingly, when patients with high blood pressure are put on a low-sodium diet, within six to eight weeks many discover that the foods they used to eat now seem unpleasantly salty.

To a degree, cravings also reflect cultural preferences. After all, a Swede is unlikely to develop a longing for tortilla chips. And to a large extent, affluence is a precondition. In societies where people face a constant struggle against starvation, cravings are virtually unknown. But when such people are exposed to a high-fat Western diet, they develop the same types of preferences as Westerners. According to Dr. Drewnowski, that's one reason fast-food restaurants are making huge inroads in the Far East.

A TASTE OF THE FUTURE

Scientists are studying ex-smokers, people with depression, athletes and those recovering from prolonged illness in an attempt to sort out the complicated physical and psychological cues that lead us to crave specific foods. The work is still new, but someday, researchers say, they hope to be able to help people satisfy all their food longings . . . and still maintain a healthy diet and optimal weight. Now that would truly be having your cake—and eating it, too.

—*Beth Weinhouse*

PART THREE

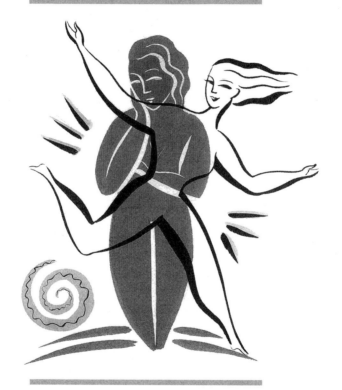

SAY GOOD-BYE
TO STRESS AND FATIGUE

STRESS BUSTERS
THAT WORK

DOZENS OF LITTLE ANNOYANCES CAN ADD UP
TO BIG-TIME STRESS. BUT GUESS WHAT?
THERE ARE DOZENS OF LITTLE WAYS
TO SEND IT PACKING.

The word alone is enough to make your shoulders hunch and your brow furrow. What your body knows instinctively is that stress—a physical response to a psychological overload—hurts. This mind/body relationship has kept researchers busy for decades.

Their findings? It's not only the big-time angst of divorce, unemployment and job change that takes a toll. It's the everyday stress of babies crying and appliances breaking down, of traffic tie-ups and late dinners that lead to stress-related health problems ranging from acne to increased risk of heart disease.

For tips on beating stress, we went to the real experts: women just like you who have learned to relax despite it all.

BEATING THE MORNING PANIC

Plan ahead. Start the night before by setting the table for breakfast and fixing lunches. Make sure you (and the kids) know what you're going to wear the next day, and check everything for missing buttons, rips and spots.

Get up early. "I get up one hour before my husband and kids do," says Connie West, a mother of four in Jasonville, Indiana. "That's my time to be by myself, to pray and to get mentally prepared for the rest of the day."

Share the load. "I help my two kids get dressed, then my husband gives them breakfast while I get dressed," says Jane Davidson, a Spanish teacher from East Northport, New York. "Those few minutes of uninterrupted time in the morning are a must."

Set the clocks ahead five to ten minutes. But don't tell anyone. You'll worry less about getting everyone off on time.

Post reminders on the door or the refrigerator. This helps ensure that you don't forget anything—like lunches, library books, special appointments.

GETTING THROUGH THE DAY MORE EASILY

Take breaks. "I make it a point to spend 15 minutes in the morning and again in the evening doing yoga and meditation," says Nancy Ellner, a social worker and part-time radio announcer in Garden City, New York. "It clears my mind of pressure and makes me more calm."

Walk more. Like other aerobic exercise, walking is a natural stress reliever. "I make regular walking dates with a friend," says Connie West. "By the time we've gone a mile and talked things out, I feel great."

Don't try to do too much at once. "When I'm feeling overwhelmed by the number of tasks that face me," says stylist Danielle DiGiacomo, "I tell myself I only have to do one—but I must do it right away. That gets me started—and before I know it, the work no longer seems overwhelming."

Try to shop and bank at off hours when lines are short. One early riser goes to the supermarket before breakfast and finishes in record time.

Have a spare umbrella. Keep one in your car, office and tote so you'll never be caught in the rain without one.

Make sure you have duplicates of important items. These include anything you'd be lost without—such as your reading glasses, bank card or list of important numbers.

Go to the bathroom before leaving anywhere. Also make sure your children do the same. That will be one less thing to worry about if you experience a delay.

Get a cordless phone. Take it with you when working in the yard or the garage—or simply relaxing. Then you won't have to dash to answer a ring.

Give yourself permission to be imperfect. Let the dust pile up, use convenience foods, give a gift certificate instead of searching for the perfect blouse for Mom.

Get a personal tape player. Then take it—and your favorite tapes—along when you expect a long wait or a stressful encounter (a dentist appointment, a rush-hour shopping trip, even a line at a popular movie).

Make sure there is a phone at any meeting place. If you're going shopping or to a movie with a friend, meet in a coffee shop instead of at the theater or the mall, where you won't be able to make contact if there's an unavoidable delay.

Devise ways to deal with stressful people. If you can't avoid them, try to maintain control of all encounters. MaryBeth Farrell, a San Francisco accountant, says, "I never ask time-wasters to sit down in my office; they may never get up. I also try to keep them from going off on tangents."

Approach things with a sense of humor. Call a friend in the middle of the day to share a joke; make a funny face at a co-worker. Search for the humor in situations when everything seems to go wrong.

Browse. One survey found that browsing in bookstores was a top stress-reducer for many women. Laurie Drake of Los Angeles does her browsing at the Farmer's Market. "Just looking at the array of colors and shapes of food—not to mention the variety of people there—is very soothing."

Learn to say "No," and "I'll get back to you." "If someone insists on an immediate answer from me," says MaryBeth Farrell, "I usually say, 'I have to call you back.' Allowing myself even ten minutes to consider a request or question helps me avoid giving wrong answers in haste."

WINDING DOWN IN THE EVENING

Invest in an answering machine. Refuse to answer the phone when you're eating or busy. "My phone always seemed to ring just as I put my baby in the tub," says Ann Zimmerman, a Dallas mother. "Now I let the machine answer, then I return calls when I'm more relaxed." A machine also lets you screen out unwanted calls from salespeople.

Put music into your life. "I sing along with the radio as I maneuver through the Boston traffic," says Judy Kennedy, an administrative assistant in West Roxbury, Massachusetts. "It helps settle my nerves."

Indulge yourself for at least a few minutes every night. "I love to settle down with a good mystery novel in the evening," says Joan Knaub, a school librarian and mother of two. Other women relax with long baths, needlepoint or other hobbies.

Get in touch with your childhood. Reread your favorite children's book. Flip through a photo album. Play a board game. "My husband and I have a running backgammon championship," says Joan Roberts of Chicago. "We play a few nights a week. It's very relaxing and helps us to keep fun in our marriage."

Watch a tear-jerker movie. "Nothing is more stress-relieving than a good cry," says Jane Davidson.

Focus on the positive. "Every night I write down in my notebook at least one pleasant thing that happened during the day," says Connie West. "It may be a compliment I received or a few minutes I spent watching a squirrel gathering nuts. Then, when everything seems to be going wrong, I pull out this journal and it puts me in a great mood."

At bedtime, thank everyone in your family for their help that day. According to Raymond Flannery, Jr., Ph.D., a stress researcher at Harvard Medical School and author of *Becoming Stress Resistant,* "It will make you feel good, make them feel appreciated and will nurture the relationships that are so important to reducing stress."

Pursue a hobby you truly enjoy. "I love to knit," says Beverly Avadikian, a grandmother from Potsdam, New York. "It's relaxing to do it, and it gives me a head start on Christmas presents, too."

Spend time with a pet. Studies show that simply petting an animal can lower blood pressure. "When I return from work, I walk my dog for half an hour," says Sheila Shulman, crafts editor for *Woman's Day* magazine. "It puts him in a great mood and makes me feel good, too."

MAKING YOUR LIFE A LITTLE EASIER

Think of delays as opportunities to reduce stress. When you're held up in a long line or a traffic jam, daydream, plan your next vacation, do soothing neck rolls or deep-breathing exercises.

Allow yourself time for mistakes. You'll be less upset by lost keys, traffic delays and other glitches if you haven't overbooked your day.

Stock up on things you don't dare run out of. These include toilet paper, paper towels, tampons, toothpaste.

Buy extra birthday cards and gifts as you see them. This way, you won't have to rush around at the last minute.

Make duplicates of all your house and car keys. Give copies to family members and a trusted neighbor.

Keep your appliances and other machines well maintained. Get regular tune-ups and oil changes on your car, for instance, to prevent untimely—and stressful—breakdowns.

Have regular medical checkups. Early detection of a serious problem can save your life. And sometimes just finding out that you're in good health can be a stress reducer.

Eliminate clutter. The more that's on your desk or in your closet, the harder it is to find what you're looking for. Take one room at a time and get rid of everything you don't need or use.

Carry spare change. Keep some in your purse, car, briefcase and pockets so you are always prepared for toll gates, parking meters, pay phones and vending machines.

Keep some extra money in accessible places. If you have a few dollars in your desk or car, for example, and your handbag is lost or stolen, you won't be totally broke.

Leave hard-to-replace items in a safe place at home. If you don't really need your checkbook, family photos, address book, credit cards and driver's license every day, why take the chance of losing them from your purse?

STRESSLESS PARENTING

Spend time away from your kids. A baby-sitter who comes after school a few times a week can make a big difference. "I joined a baby-sitting co-op with other mothers in my daughter's class," says Jean Poole of West Hills, California. "That gives me an occasional afternoon to myself—and Michelle gets to spend more time with her friends."

Share advice with other mothers. "I'm in a bowling league," says Jean Poole. "We bowl, sip coffee and share parenting stories. It's the best stress reducer in my week."

Try not to take things personally. "I used to get upset when my 15-year-old talked fresh," says Carol O'Grady. "Now I remind myself that all kids misbehave from time to time. When mine act up occasionally, it's not a direct reflection on me."

Play outside with your kids occasionally. Shooting baskets, skating, jumping rope and other active games can relieve stress and make you feel closer to your children.

—*Laura Flynn McCarthy*

HOW TO GET RID OF THAT TIRED FEELING

IT'S OFTEN THE QUALITY, NOT THE QUANTITY, OF YOUR SLEEP THAT LEAVES YOU FEELING OUT OF SORTS THE NEXT DAY. WITH A LITTLE PRACTICE, YOU CAN LEARN HOW TO IMPROVE THE WAY YOU SLEEP—AND THE WAY YOU FEEL.

The last time you felt draggy or irritable, chances are you vowed to start getting more sleep. But snoozing longer isn't always the solution to daytime drowsiness. While most of us think that "how much" is the only important variable affecting our nightly slumber, more and more research is finding that quantity is only half the story. Sleep quality, which has long been given short shrift, is just as important to our physical and mental well-being, says Charles Pollak, M.D., head of the Sleep/Wake Disorders Center at the New York Hospital—Cornell Medical Center in White Plains, New York.

"People often couch their sleep complaints in terms of how much they get, when the real nature of their problem happens to lie in the way they sleep," Dr. Pollak says.

"Poor sleep is an almost universal phenomenon," he notes. Recent studies have shown that many of the realities of modern life, ranging from stress overload to poor diet to a noisy environment, can lead to shallow, fragmented sleep. And we pay a high price for poor sleeping habits. A recent report from the National Commission on Sleep Disorders Research found that inadequate slumber costs the nation $16 billion per year, resulting from sleep-related accidents and lost or inefficient work time.

The good news from the frontiers of sleep science is that researchers have now identified some ways to help us sleep better, and these new strategies have the potential to produce more restful nights and brighter days for all of us.

POOR SLUMBER TAKES ITS TOLL

Those with severe insomnia know they have a problem, but many people may not be aware of subtle sleep deficits. A common tip-off to inadequate slumber is an inability to handle dull or repetitive tasks. "If you're taking an important exam or going on a job interview, you'll probably do all right," Dr. Pollak says. "But you'll have problems if you have to type a detailed report, drive a long distance or balance your checkbook."

Another sign of substandard sleep: "Your ability to organize information and think things through carefully may be impaired," says Timothy M. Monk, Ph.D., a psychologist and the director of the Human-Chronobiology Program at the University of Pittsburgh. If you're taking care of young children, for example, you may have trouble coordinating their activities.

But perhaps the highest price of sleepiness is that it leaves you irritable. Your temper is shorter, and you're apt to be edgy and therefore less pleasant to family members and co-workers. (To assess your sleep quality, see "How Well Are You Sleeping?" on page 107.)

Women's moods may be particularly vulnerable to poor sleep, says Kathryn Lee, Ph.D., an assistant professor in the School of Nursing at the University of California, San Francisco. She has found that women susceptible to premenstrual syndrome—which includes irritability, fatigue and anxiety—get shallow sleep all month long. Their underlying fatigue may make it harder to handle hormonal changes. "If women with PMS work on increasing their deep sleep throughout the month, they might be able to alleviate their symptoms," Dr. Lee says. (See the tips that follow.)

In the past, experts trying to help us sleep better were limited by a lack of understanding about how slumber works. The only way to study sleep was to awaken people and ask them questions—a method that yielded little meaningful information. However, sophisticated machines now allow scientists to record bodily functions, particularly brain waves, while subjects remain asleep. As a result, researchers now know what good sleep consists of, and they've identified the culprits that interfere with sound slumber.

THE SLEEP ROBBERS

Sleep should progress continuously through four stages. The final stage is REM sleep—a term that stands for "rapid eye movement," which takes place when the brain suddenly ignites with dreams. Each night we should go through the complete cycle about four or five times with few interruptions.

It's normal to wake up briefly two to ten times per night due to things like shifting around to stay comfortable, but some of us awaken more frequently. This may fragment sleep and make us spend an inordinate amount of time in the lightest, least-refreshing stages. In fact, researchers found being awakened briefly every ten minutes throughout the night had the same sleep-robbing effect as a three- to four-hour sleep loss (though we may not remember our awakenings).

"The degree to which you're sleepy during the day is directly related to how often you're aroused at night," says psychologist Timothy Roehrs, Ph.D., director of research at the Sleep Disorders Center at Henry Ford Hospital in Detroit.

Noise—from a child's cry, planes flying overhead or automobile traffic, for example—is a common source of interruption. In fact, studies have shown that most people who live near airports or busy streets never fully adjust to the racket. Mental arousal and worry can also wreak havoc with sleep.

A case in point: Medical and railroad workers who are on call spend less time in the deeper stages of sleep and feel more tired when they wake up than when they're not on call. In addition, sleep can suffer when something disrupts our daily, or circadian, rhythms, which include body temperature, metabolic rate and hormone levels. Various indicators of time, such as the onset of daylight and the time we get up, keep these rhythms synchronized. If they are thrown off, by sleeping in on weekends, for example, your sleep may become more shallow and you may have difficulty falling asleep in the first place.

HOW TO REST EASY

The following slumber strategies can counteract common sleep spoilers. (If you have persistent insomnia or daytime drowsiness, see your physician.)

Set your biological clock. To keep your circadian rhythms in sync, go to bed and wake up at the same time each day. "The minute you alter your sleep schedule, you reduce your quality of sleep," Dr. Roehrs says. Also, try to get a generous dose of early morning light. Ideally you should spend about 45 minutes outdoors.

Adjust your internal thermostat. Doing something to raise your body temperature in the late afternoon will cause it to fall at bedtime, making your sleep deeper, says Peter Hauri, Ph.D., a clinical psychologist and administrative director of the Mayo Clinic Sleep Disorders Center in Rochester, Minnesota. Dr. Hauri recommends walking briskly, swimming or engaging in any other activity that boosts your heart and breathing rate for 20 minutes. (Working out in the early morning has no effect on sleep, while exercising within three hours of bedtime can keep you awake.) Soaking in a hot bath for about 20 minutes an hour or two before bedtime can also raise body temperature and improve sleep.

Keep your bedroom at a comfortable temperature. Some studies have indicated that sleep becomes more fragmented when the room temperature goes above 75° or falls below 68°.

Turn down the volume. If you live near an airport or busy street, you can minimize noise by padding floors with thick carpeting, covering windows with heavy drapes and investing in soundproof windows. In addition, you can block unwanted sounds by wearing earplugs or drown out noise with a fan, an air conditioner or a white-noise machine.

Synchronize family sleep schedules. If your child's early-morning awakenings hinder your sleep, consider adjusting her sleep regimen. Make her bedtime, mealtimes and naptimes about ten minutes later every day until she's on the desired schedule. Do the reverse if your child's slumber routine runs later than you'd like.

If your child wakes you up in the middle of the night, you can make up for lost slumber by sleeping in an hour later or by catching a short nap in the afternoon.

Get the right vitamins. Women tend to be deficient in

HOW WELL ARE YOU SLEEPING?

If you experience any of these problems during the day, you may need better-quality sleep.
- You find yourself rereading the same paragraph.
- You nod off during church services or a movie.
- You have trouble with concentrating, remembering things, following complex tasks through to the end or organizing information.
- You have difficulty listening to other people's point of view.

a number of nutrients important to high-quality sleep. Normal levels of iron, for example, keep you from waking at night, while copper (which many people may be deficient in) helps you fall asleep, says James Penland, Ph.D., a research psychologist at the U.S. Department of Agriculture Human Nutrition Research Center in Grand Forks, North Dakota. He's found in studies that women who got the Recommended Dietary Allowance (RDA) of these minerals slept better than those who got one-third of that amount. Some sources of iron and copper include low-fat beef, poultry, fish, green vegetables and whole grains.

Women taking birth control pills are often deficient in vitamin B_6, which helps produce serotonin, a brain chemical that calms people and makes them sleepy. If you're on the Pill, make sure you get at least the RDA of vitamin B_6. (Chicken, fish, potatoes and whole grains are good sources.)

Eat plenty of carbohydrates. Like vitamin B_6, these nutrients promote the manufacture of serotonin, says Judith J. Wurtman, Ph.D., a research scientist in the Department of Brain and Cognitive Science at the Massachusetts Institute of Technology in Cambridge. Women on liquid diets or on quick-loss diets that forbid breads and cereals may lack carbs, resulting in shallow sleep. Experts recommend that people take in a least four servings of carbohydrates a day. Also, never go to bed hungry; this may interfere with sleep.

Prevent stomach upsets. Avoid some other foods, at least in the evening. "This includes anything you know is a gastric irritant for you," says psychologist James Walsh, Ph.D., past president of the American Sleep Disorders Association. "If you eat spicy food before bed, you may frequently awaken from reflux material [stomach acid backwashing into your esophagus]. It may feel like heartburn, or you might awaken without feeling discomfort."

Banish worry from the bedroom. "The best thing scientists could do to improve sleep would be to invent a system for not thinking," advises sleep researcher Wilse Webb, Ph.D., of the University of Florida in Gainesville. One way to keep daytime worries from intruding into your night is to complete personal business early in the evening, leaving the two hours before bedtime free for calming activities such as reading or watching TV. But if your problems continue to haunt you, try writing down your troubles, noting a solution next to each one. Regular physical activity and relaxation exercises, such as deep breathing, can also reduce nighttime worries. If you can't fall asleep in less than a half hour, don't continue to toss and turn in bed. Go into another room and do a quiet activity until you're drowsy.

Skip the nightcap. Contrary to popular belief, drinking alcoholic beverages will make you sleep worse, not better. In tests, Dr. Roehrs discovered that people who had several drinks before bed slept very deeply during the first part of the night, while the alcohol was metabolizing, but the rest of their sleep was so shallow that the next day their reaction times dropped by 10 percent. Experts recommend limiting your evening intake to one drink at least two hours before turning in. If you're at a party and plan to have a couple of drinks, stop imbibing four to five hours before bedtime to avoid sleep disturbance.

Stay away from stimulants. Caffeine can cause insomnia and poor-quality sleep. To keep it from having any effect on your slumber, don't consume any beverages that contain caffeine after 2 P.M.

Many pills impair sleep as well, including diet pills, over-the-counter decongestants and pain relievers containing caffeine; don't take them less than four hours before going to sleep. Prescription sleeping pills may help you sleep at first, but they may lose their effectiveness and become addictive after a few weeks. Also, once you stop taking them, you may have even more trouble falling asleep.

Avoid lingering in bed. While studies show many of us don't get enough sleep, some people may snooze too much. Staying in bed excessively long or napping too much can make sleep shallower and more fragmented. Never nap for longer than one hour or after 4 P.M.; either can make you less sleepy at bedtime, says Dr. Webb.

—*Richard Laliberte*

PART FOUR

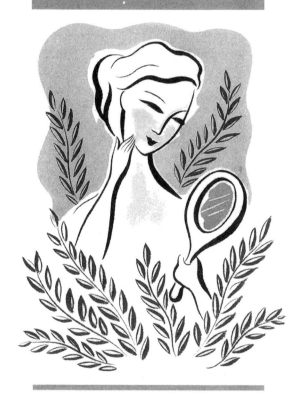

LOOKING GOOD

FOREVER
YOUNGER SKIN

RESTORING THE BLOOM OF YOUTH IS BECOMING
LESS OF A PIPE DREAM AND MORE OF A POSSIBILITY,
AS SCIENTISTS DISCOVER NEW WAYS TO COMBAT
AGING AND PRESERVE SKIN'S RESILIENCE.

What happens when you play billiards and the cue hits a cluster of balls? They scatter and lose energy. That's exactly what happens when the UVA and UVB rays in sunlight hit the melanin in human skin. They scatter and have less energy, less detrimental effect. Ergo, the more melanin in the skin, the more it is protected. This is the reason, of course, that black skin, with much more melanin than white skin, ages less and is less susceptible to skin cancer." It is 10 A.M. in New York and biochemist Sergio Nacht, Ph.D., is calling from the Advanced Polymer System (APS) lab in Redwood City, California, where at 7 A.M. he has already put in an hour's work.

For scientists like Dr. Nacht on the brink of more than one skin-saving discovery, it isn't difficult these days to work more and sleep less. Today Dr. Nacht is describing, in his usual unorthodox but enlightening way, his company's lead in the race to find a synthetic melanin to mimic exactly the pigment that both colors and protects human skin. Years of genetic engineering research have gone into the project, years of studying the melanin in cuttlefish, black caviar, squid and mushrooms, years of trying to formulate a light brown melanin suitable for use in a cream.

"Whether it will be a prescription drug or an over-the-counter product, the FDA will decide. One thing we do know is that this cream will provide all skins with the most complete protection ever available, not only because of the additional melanin but also because of the Microsponge delivery system we are using, which will also carry sunscreen," says Dr. Nacht.

REVERSING THE AGING PROCESS

The Microsponge, patented by Advanced Polymer Systems in 1987, is the most precise system of delivering drugs to the skin. Soon, as the result of a unique multimillion-dollar contract signed with Ortho, the makers of Retin-A, the Microsponge will be used in the most advanced skin care for treating acne and photoaging.

Dr. Nacht describes it like this: "Imagine a talcum powder in which each particle is a sponge about 25 microns in diameter—that's one one-thousandth of an inch. A substance is loaded into each sponge and with a time-release mechanism is very slowly disseminated. A gram, which is the usual dosage, contains about a hundred million Microsponges. The Microsponge is the perfect way to minimize side effects when using potent formulas."

One of the most potent is tretinoin (Retin-A), a controversial substance ever since the news broke in the mid-1980s that it appeared to be able to reverse signs of aging in skin. In the spring of 1992, several of the most illustrious names in the world of dermatology, as members of a special FDA advisory board, held up their hands to signal their unanimous recommendation for tretinoin, in a cream to be called Renova, to be used to treat the fine wrinkling, hyperpigmentation and roughness associated with photodamaged (prematurely aged) skin. Renova would become the first topical antiaging drug.

Arnold Schroeter, M.D., chairman of the Department of Dermatology at Wright State University School of Medicine in Dayton, Ohio; Jonathon Wilkin, M.D., director of the Department of Dermatology at Ohio State University in Columbus; and Joseph McGuire, Jr., M.D., professor of dermatology at the Stanford University Medical Center in California, were among those who voted, but the historic decision didn't make waves—only CNN made a special announcement on its "Headline News."

Perhaps it was because the favorable vote come as no surprise; also perhaps because there are so many trenchant skin-care advances today that address what the *British Journal of Plastic Surgery* once described as "the disfigurement of the aging face . . . a triad of hollow, sag and wrinkle." At that time, in the seventies, it was believed that the only way to rid the face of fine wrinkles was to use an acid peel of phenol to destroy the skin's top layer, "burning out the wrinkle" by changing the cellular construction beneath to collapse vertical age lines.

HIGH-TECH MIRACLES FOR THE SKIN

Today, instead of phenol, a new star ingredient, glycolic acid (derived from sugar cane), is being used by physicians to peel away fine lines. Many doctors are combining glycolic acid peels with carefully monitored Retin-A treatments and sunscreens, a combo described by Melvin Elson, M.D., a Nashville dermatologist, as "a skin rejuvenation program." In his own research centers in Tennessee and New York, Dr. Elson, like many dermatologists today, both evaluates and helps formulate products in professional and over-the-counter strengths to treat prematurely aged skin. The professional peeling product (called M.D. Formulations, which Dr. Elson helped created with Herald Pharmacal), contains 70 percent glycolic acid and is used every 2 weeks over a 12-week period. The products for home use—cleaners and moisturizers—contain 40 percent glycolic acid. Dr. Elson also prescribes a low-dose Retin-A cream at night and sunscreen every day, sun or no sun.

He explains the effects of the treatment: "You know when steam from the shower fogs up the bathroom mirror and you can't see a thing? You wipe it off so you can see again. That's what a glycolic acid peel does—it wipes the slate clean on the outer skin to give it a totally fresh start. Using the peels in conjunction with Retin-A doubles the fresh effect."

Glycolic acid is but one of a group of nontoxic alphahydroxy acids (AHAs) that are being used increasingly in skin-care products. When James J. Leyden, M.D., professor of dermatology at the University of Pennsylvania in Philadelphia, spoke about AHAs, he explained their relevance to Retin-A this way: "AHAs were first recognized for their ability to draw moisture to the skin, but they're much more than moisturizers. In using them on dry, thickened, sun-damaged skin, we saw a remarkable change—to a thin, compact layer that looked and felt better. We thought the thinning effect would make the stratum corneum [the skin's outer layer] more vulnerable to irritants, but the opposite was true. We developed a new hypothesis: AHA molecules thin the stratum corneum but also make it more resilient. We then realized it would be good for dermatologists to prescribe them in conjunction with Retin-A treatments to diminish irritating side effects.

"As further evidence that AHAs are much more than moisturizers, my colleagues and I at the University of Pennsylvania have just published studies in the *Journal of the American Academy of Dermatology* that show that AHAs cut the negative effects of cortisone creams by 50 percent. They also have an effect on brittle nails, so we'll see AHA products in that area, too.

"We're only now getting a sense of their potential application. If the eighties were the Retin-A decade, the next ten years will be devoted to AHAs."

The latest research has also lead to the use of glycolic acid in a gel formulated with hydroquinone, an FDA-approved skin-lightening drug, to lighten freckles and age and sun spots. Howard Murad, M.D., an assistant clinical professor of dermatology at UCLA, is the brains behind this advance.

Avon is the first major company to use glycolic acid in a strengthening, firming skin-care treatment, Anew Perfecting Complex for Face, the most successful treatment product in Avon's 106-year history. They also have Anew Perfecting Complex for Chest and Neck (areas often more damaged by the sun, Dr. Leyden states, than the face) and Vertical Lip Line Smoothing Cream with glycolic acid and vitamin A to help rid the lip area of wrinkles, into which lipstick often "bleeds," ruining its effect.

With the introduction of Formule Intensive Day Lift Refining Complex, Chanel is using glycolic acid in its own patent-pending formula, which promises to tackle poor skin texture and discoloration.

U.S. patent no. 4,138,479 protects the processing of the other superstar natural ingredient of the nineties, a yeast extract known as Nayad. The patent was purchased from Bayer in 1985 by Texas entrepreneur Byron Donzis for his ImmuDyne company.

YEASTS AND PETROLEUM JELLY

Nayad has been described in many ways: as a component of yeast that's a distant cousin to the active ingredient in Preparation H; more attractively as the same ingredient that makes the breakfast spreads Marmite and Vegemite so tasty to British and Australian palates. Technically, however, Nayad is a beta glucan, an active chemical extracted from the cellular wall of baker's yeast, which ImmuDyne's research suggests can speed the healing of wounds and the repair of sun-damaged skin by restoring weakened collagen and elastic fibers, the root cause of sag and wrinkles. Not surprisingly, this research has stimulated the interest of major cosmetics companies like Elizabeth Arden, which introduced Nayad into its Immunage UV Defense line, and of smaller specialized lines like Elysée.

Walter P. Smith, Ph.D., former director of research and development for Estée Lauder, recently developed a mail-order Nayad-based skin-care line for ImmuDyne—Nayad now comes in three strengths—and soon Nayad will be a major ingredient in Yves St. Laurent's new Precursor skin-care line to fortify and revitalize damaged skin.

Even petroleum jelly is having a new day with a recent announcement from the American Academy of Dermatology. Through a new chemical-fixing process that provides very clear pictures of changes to the skin's intercellular layers, it could be seen that petrolatum not only acts as a protective coating, it also penetrates to every level of the stratum corneum and actually helps damaged skin to repair itself.

Few people write about aging in all its many aspects with more insight and clarity than one of the most eminent men in medicine, Lewis Thomas, M.D., now president emeritus of the Memorial Sloan-Kettering Cancer Center in New

York City. In his most recent book, *The Fragile Species,* in the chapter "The Odds on Normal Aging," he writes, "There has never been a period of such high excitement and exuberance and confidence in any field of biology . . . The virologists are having a perpetual field day; the immunologists are ready to claim the whole problem of cancer as well as aging as their own; the biophysicists, the nucleic acid chemists, the geneticists, the cell biologists are falling all over each other in the race to final answers . . . Probably we will soon discover why a normal cell becomes an aging cell."

Then perhaps forever younger will become reality.

—*Shirley Lord*

THE BAD THINGS WOMEN DO IN THE NAME OF GOOD SKIN

MANY BEAUTY REGIMENS CAN LEAD TO BREAK-OUTS, RASHES OR EVEN WORSE. HERE'S HOW TO AVOID THE MOST COMMON SKIN-CARE MISTAKES.

In the quest for perfect skin, many women create more problems than they solve. The good news: Most damage can be prevented by adopting a simpler skin-care routine. You can do your face a favor by avoiding these beauty blunders.

Overmoisturizing. "Many women believe they'll wrinkle faster if they don't use a moisturizer, so they slather it on even if they have oily skin," says D'Anne Kleinsmith, M.D., staff dermatologist at William Beaumont Hospital near Detroit. In fact, moisturizers can't prevent wrinkles, although they may minimize their appearance. (Some moisturizers contain sunscreen, which is the only bona fide anti-wrinkle ingredient.) The problem is that moisturizers, especially heavy ones, can plug pores in oily skin, causing white-heads. Overmoisturizing can also lead to seborrheic dermatitis, in which oil glands become irritated and skin peels and flakes. "People assume the flaking is from dryness, when it's really from inflamed oil glands. They keep piling on moisturizers, and the skin keeps getting worse," says New Orleans dermatologist Nia Terezakis, M.D. "What they should do is stay away from any kind of cream or lotion."

If your skin isn't acne-prone, a moisturizer probably won't do you any harm. But skip it in places where your skin is even a little oily.

Eye-cream overkill. Heavy eye creams and other greasy cosmetics (such as petroleum jelly or concealers) can cause outbreaks of milia—white cysts about the size of a pinhead—which are common in women in their thirties and forties, says New York dermatologist Ellen Gendler, M.D. If you lay off the creams, the milia may go away by themselves; if not, a dermatologist can remove them.

Almost no one needs cream on eyelid skin, which is richly supplied with oil glands. You may wish to use a light eye cream on undereye skin if it feels dry, but tiny lines around the eyes won't be helped by any cream, says Dr. Terezakis—they're caused by sun and age, not dryness.

Incorrect cleansing. Conventional wisdom has it that rich cleansing creams and milks are better for skin than soap. Emollient cleansers do feel good, and you probably need them if you wear oil-based makeup. But creamy cleansers may leave oily residues that can cause blackheads and white-heads, so be sure to rinse with warm water until all traces of cleanser are removed.

Dermatologists agree that mild soap is the best cleanser—and that it's a myth that soap dries skin. "Soap may remove some surface oils and temporarily change skin's pH level so it feels tight for 15 to 20 minutes. But it quickly returns to normal," says dermatologist Stuart M. Brown, M.D., clinical professor of dermatology at the University of Texas Health Science Center in Dallas. If the tight feeling bothers you, pat skin dry and apply a light moisturizer outside the T-zone (the forehead, nose and chin area, where oil glands tend to be larger and more active). Or try a mild soap-free cleanser like Cepaphil, Lubriderm One-Step or Oil of Olay Foaming Face Wash. If you have oily or acne-prone skin, you may wish to use a toner after cleansing to temporarily blot excess oil.

Too much scrubbing. Many of us believe our skin will look better if we exfoliate: slough off dead surface cells to reveal "new" skin underneath. Actually, skin does this all by itself, though using a mild, nongritty facial scrub once a week or so can leave it feeling smoother. Problems arise when scrubbing is taken to extremes. "I see many women whose cheeks are red and scaly from gritty scrubs or skin brushes, which leave skin with tiny scratches," says Joseph P. Bark, M.D., a Lexington, Kentucky, dermatologist.

"Women who have acne often think it's because their skin's not clean enough, so they exfoliate every day, causing irritation and inflammation," says Dr. Gendler. If your skin is extra sensitive—to the point where even a rub with a towel causes redness—avoid scrubbing altogether.

Steam "cleaning." Contrary to popular belief, steaming your face does not open pores; it actually swells them shut by plumping up cells in the skin's top layer. Steaming will make pimples worse (that's why the worst acne erupts in hot, humid climates). "I've had acne patients come in with a sudden explosion of whiteheads, and it turns out they've recently bought a facial sauna," says Dr. Bark. If you don't have acne, steaming won't hurt your skin, but it won't make it easier to remove "impurities" either.

Mask mismanagement. Most masks are harmless, but some can be trouble. Avoid gel masks that harden and get peeled off: Tiny bits of gel can remain in pores, plugging oil glands and creating major breakouts. "The plugs will work their way out eventually, but not without causing whiteheads and acne," says Dr. Bark. Soft masks that wash off are usually not a problem. Use them if you like the way your skin feels afterward—just be sure to rinse thoroughly.

Over-the-counter overload. Hoping to thwart breakouts, many women buy the strongest over-the-counter acne medication they can find—10 percent benzoyl peroxide—and wind up with red, burning skin. "Benzoyl peroxide is a good product, but it's also very harsh," says Dr. Brown. "Unless your skin is very oily—the oil provides a buffer against irritation—start with a lower concentration (2.5 to 5 percent) and gradually build to a stronger one."

Another common mistake is using drugstore medicines for long periods or on breakouts that won't be helped by them. "If over-the-counter medications don't clear up mild acne within a few weeks, see a dermatologist," says Dr. Bark. Such medications won't help red bumps or under-the-skin cysts, which require doctor-prescribed antibiotics.

The big squeeze. Squeezing whiteheads—or any blemish tinged with red—can lead to infection. "As you squeeze the top off, you push the rest of the inflammation downward," says Dr. Terezakis. "If you leave it alone, it'll usually go away much faster."

Ditto for other minor skin imperfections. "What most women call blackheads are actually enlarged pores," says Seattle dermatologist Ivor Caro, M.D. "These may have little sebum plugs—that's common on oily areas of skin—but they're not blemishes." Squeezing them can produce inflammation and scarring. It's also useless, because the pores will refill within a day or two.

Even women who leave their blemishes alone may let a salon facialist squeeze them. Bad idea: That can lead to scarring or other, more serious complications.

"Sometimes what appear to be whiteheads are actually flat warts," says Dr. Terezakis. "A facialist may squeeze these by mistake, spreading the wart virus—and new warts—all over the face." Herpes outbreaks can be mistaken for pimples and spread in the same way.

Surplus sunscreen. Wearing sunscreen daily is one of the best things you can do for your skin. But layering on more than one—putting on, say, an SPF foundation over an SPF moisturizer—can cause redness, irritation and clogged pores in women who are sensitive to sunblocks' active ingredients. "Women who get sudden outbreaks of these symptoms should suspect their sunscreens if they've recently started using more than one at a time," says Dr. Gendler. "An SPF 15 moisturizer worn with a non-SPF foundation should give them the protection they need without the irritation."

—*Marcia Menter*

MEGATRENDS
IN FASHION

IT USED TO BE THAT WOMEN SLAVISHLY FOLLOWED RULES DICTATED BY THE GREAT FASHION HOUSES. NOW WOMEN ARE TELLING THE FASHION MOGULS WHAT THEY WANT.

Financial planners say women spend too much money on clothing. But for those who really love clothes, fashion is more about creativity than logic. Fashion for some women is a leisure-time activity, somewhat like spectator sports are for men. Like sports, it gets extensive media coverage. While he pores over the sports page, she might thumb through *Vogue*, *Mirabella* or *Elle*. Many a woman considers looking at fashion the ideal way to spend a Saturday with her best friend.

Fashion is a woman's ready muse in the quest for self-expression. It is her wardrobe mistress in the drama of corporate success. But if fashion is to support a woman's success and satisfaction, it must come from the inside out. When a woman's clothing accurately reflects her taste and style and flatters her body type, something clicks psychologically. She feels empowered to take on the world.

Fashion trends are a barometer of social change. In 1851 Amelia Bloomer introduced loose-fitting harem pants or bloomers, but they did not become popular until bicycles became the rage in the Gay Nineties. Coco Chanel introduced "yachting pants" in the 1920s, but, says *The Encyclopaedia of Fashion*, "The real pants revolution came in the 1960s." Notice how the twenties are associated with women's suffrage and the sixties with the women's movement.

Much as women insist they love pants for comfort, "Numerous studies have shown that the surge in pantswear corresponded to the more or less conscious desire on the part of most women to affirm their equality with men by dressing like them"—so says *Twenty Thousand Years of Fashion: The History of Costume and Personal Adornment.*

Today's fashion, and the retail industry that sells it, reflect the shift from an industrial to an information society—which brought millions of women into the workplace. That megashift revved up the retail industry: Millions of women needed new work clothes and had the income to buy them.

The "Dress for Success" look, that pseudomale costume of a dark suit and tie, made sense when women first entered the work force 20 years ago. Now that women are a critical mass in business and the professions, a new cadre of female designers, led by Donna Karan, are devoted to dressing customers comfortably, elegantly—and like women. "As a woman, my understanding of it is unique," says Karan. Male designers once ruled Seventh Avenue. No longer. Today Liz Claiborne generates almost four times the women's clothing sales of the top three male designers combined.

DESIGNING WOMEN

Today 53 million women need something to wear to work. Though affluent, they are in no position to afford clothing with a couture pricetag. Top designers are following the lead of Anne Klein II, the first house to successfully launch a major "secondary line" of well-designed, moderately priced collections that bear the designer's name.

At odds with the financial advisers, who say, "Put the money you spend on clothes into tax-free bonds," are career experts, who say, "Dress for the job you want, not the one you have." It is an interesting conflict. Can one justify spending more money on clothes as a career investment?

The movement of women over 40 into positions of corporate and political leadership will revolutionize fashion and retailing. As presidents of their own firms and corporate vice presidents, fortysomething women will be the first generation to define and perfect the female executive image of elegance and authority. A Donna Karan ad that ran in spring 1992 portrayed a beautiful woman running for and being elected to the U.S. presidency. Karan knew just how to dress her. (But, Donna, next time how about a gorgeous 50-year-old instead of a 30-year-old?)

DRESSING THE NEW WOMAN

The aging of the baby boom and the widening of its collective waistline are compelling designers to offer more options for women size 16 and up. Retailers, who are losing sales to catalogs, TV shopping and outlet malls, must find new ways to sell to time-conscious and price-conscious working women.

The multibillion-dollar fashion and beauty industry—and the fashion media that cover it—have a new customer. Its success in a postfeminist, postmaterialist 1990s is dependent on the ability to recognize and fulfill her changing needs. For centuries fashion and beauty set the trends top-down. A generation of now-mature male designers honed their skills dressing the ladies who lunch and attend society benefits. Wealthy matrons loyally followed their every fashion dictum.

Today's new female consumer will have none of that. She is educated, experienced, confident, affluent yet cost-conscious. *The most basic megatrend in the fashion arena is the shift from top-down to bottom-up.*

The days when women followed fashion *blindly* are over; even the industry recognizes that. The new question is: Will women "follow" fashion *at all?* Our answer is a resounding *no.* Fashion will have to start following women.

—*Patricia Aburdene and John Naisbitt*

PART FIVE

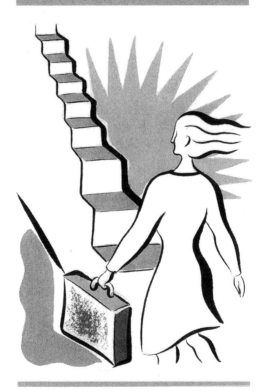

ON THE JOB

FITTING IN AT WORK

NOTHING WILL BOOST YOUR CHANCES FOR SUCCESS LIKE ADAPTING YOUR STYLE TO THE CORPORATE CULTURE AT YOUR OFFICE.

When I was growing up, one of my favorite games was Office. My best girlfriend and I played it in the upstairs hall of my parents' house. Two end tables served as desks. We were both secretaries. Neither of us wanted to play boss and hand out orders. Like our games of Dress-Up, Office was practice for the future. We weren't interested in flights of pure fancy; we wanted to try out the real roles we expected to have as adults. And from occasional visits to our fathers' offices, we knew what women did there. Their place in the business culture of the day was to take orders, not give them; their attitude was cheerful, smiling and friendly.

Since then, offices and the cultures within them have gotten a lot more complicated. Women are not limited to the bottom of the pecking order; they are all over the place, including the top. They hand out orders as well as receive them—even in my father's office. Success is no longer a simple matter of being the fastest stenographer. It involves power lunches and strategy sessions and a whole carload of skills and expertise that never came up back in the days when I was playing Office.

MY, HOW TIMES HAVE CHANGED

Women nowadays not only have an ever-growing range of choices about where they can be and what they can do. They also have a range of choices about how they can act. The old order of the day—women should be friendly and cheerful no matter what—is useless at best, and sometimes downright dangerous.

With a whole world of challenges in front of us, we can't get by any longer just letting a smile be our umbrella. We need a full repertoire of responses, starting with what to do when the situation—as it usually does—calls for a lot more than a smile.

But don't take my word for it. Let's get down to cases. Let's get down to what happened when someone who once played Office ventured out into the world still clinging to the idea that if you can't say something nice, don't say anything at all. In short, let's get down to me.

I was nervous my first few days at the major national publishing company I'll call XYZ. It was the first large concern I'd been at, and I wasn't sure how well I'd fit in. Then I met Betsy and Marilyn and liked them immediately. The new office where I would be working as an editor had seemed alien and intimidating, but not to worry. Here were friendly, reassuring faces—what luck they were there. I would just be one of the gang.

And I was, for the next six months. Every day, I did the work I was assigned, then spent the balance of my time talking to Betsy and Marilyn. Some days we chatted almost non-stop. It was a lot of fun.

Then Betsy and Marilyn moved to a different office. I was alone. For the first time, I saw what was going on around me. It didn't make me feel good. Without the distraction of Betsy and Marilyn, I couldn't help noticing that the assignments I wanted weren't coming my way. I always seemed to be the last to know what was going on. When I suggested a project, nobody listened. Slowly but surely, I got the picture: I was out of the loop.

FOLLOWING THE RIGHT SET OF RULES

For the life of me, I couldn't figure out why. I'd done my job. I hadn't missed any days; my duties were done on time; I had neat handwriting. People were glad to see me and laughed at my jokes and seemed to like me. How could there be a problem? I'd followed all the rules.

Which was, of course, precisely the problem. I had followed all the rules—but they were the wrong ones. I hadn't been hired to be friendly and cheerful and smile a lot; I'd been hired to be an editor. Unlike in earlier positions on smaller publications, where being able to make close, warm friendships quickly had been vital, I was now in a large, formal, corporate workplace. How people acted, what they expected, how they evaluated what I did—that is, their culture—was based on different needs and standards. And if I wanted to make it here, I would have to find out what they were.

I'd already made the first breakthrough: I'd figured out that they did things differently at XYZ. I didn't understand what the new rules were, but I could see that my usual approach just wouldn't wash. Faced with an unfamiliar, unwritten system that I didn't expect and didn't know how to operate in, I was disoriented and bewildered. I didn't know it at the time, but what I was feeling was really a sort of culture shock.

And appropriately so, according to Dee Soder, Ph.D., president of Endymion Company, an executive advisory firm. "Any new workplace is like a foreign land," she says, "and you have to treat it that way. Every place has its own way of doing things, and very few people fit in automatically. When you walk in, you just have to be observant and pick up on cues."

Easier said than done, of course. I was picking up on cues, but they weren't the ones that counted. Everyone—my various bosses, the personnel office, new colleagues—had told me what a pleasant place this would be to work in, how friendly the people were and how low-key. All of which was true; what they didn't mention was that getting ahead was not a function of friendliness. What distinguished those who were on their way up wasn't how pleasant they were—this was taken for granted—but how well they did everything else.

Take, for example, their attitude toward what they were doing. The editors who were getting promoted didn't just do what they were given; they were constantly on the lookout for what else they could accomplish. They studied the field, attended seminars, stayed current with the competition.

They made it clear that they wanted to learn, to grow, to get better at their job. They combed publications for promising writers and circulated ambitious memos and took home thick stacks of manuscripts to edit. They were always enthusiastic and upbeat.

Even more elementary, they didn't come to work late, like me, and they didn't look like they still hadn't woken up, again like me. Bright-eyed and bushy-tailed, they arrived early and had memos on others' desks while I was still brushing my teeth. Since the editor-in-chief was also an early bird, this gave them abundant opportunity for the sort of relaxed, informal conversation with the boss that I never seemed to have.

CLAIMING CREDIT THAT'S DUE

The rest of the day, too, they weren't waiting around to be noticed. When they did something, they put their names on it. A new author, an important article, a particularly well-done column—these didn't just somehow materialize out of the ether. The editors who were responsible took visible credit. When I got a compliment on my work, I automatically sloughed it off: "Oh, it was nothing," I'd say, regardless of how much effort I might have put into it. When one of the other editors received some praise, they not only said "thanks," but described just how hard they had to work to achieve this result. They took pride in what they'd done. Further, if they'd done a lot of work on something and nobody noticed, they brought it up. They didn't assume everyone knew what they'd done; they made sure everyone knew.

But perhaps most telling, they didn't try to make friends with everyone there. Don't get me wrong; they weren't antisocial. They were nice, they made small talk and occasional jokes, they offered congratulations and condolences when appropriate. But the relationships they had there seemed based far less on intimate confidences than on shared responsibilities and helping each other with their work.

They would mention that they'd had a nice weekend,

perhaps the name of a movie they'd seen—but not whom they went with and the exact state of their relationship to that person in full, gory detail.

Although they went through the usual life crises—kids were born, parents died, marriages broke up—they didn't use the office as a therapy center. During the rough patches in my own life, I would spend days leaning on the nearest shoulder, but other editors seemed to keep their home life out of their office life. The two were not identical; indeed, there was not even much overlap.

In short, they respected and liked their colleagues, but they did not love them. They maintained a certain distance; they held back. Which was, to me, a truly mind-boggling concept. Wasn't I supposed to pour out all my feelings, or at least try to do so? Wasn't it dishonest not to say everything that was on my mind?

Well, no, it's not. Or so I concluded after a lot of thinking and watching and talking to friends who worked in other offices. You don't have to say it all; you're not expected to. The goal of an office is to get the job done, not to probe everyone's personality in microdetail. In fact, if you're working hard enough on the job, there really isn't time for that kind of minute examination.

You don't have to lie; in fact, you shouldn't, ever. But you can decide how much to say, and to whom. There are other people involved, with their own expectations and needs and requirements. Automatically dumping on them whatever is on your mind isn't, as I had once thought, the only decent way to be. Listening to them and finding out what their concerns are is just as important, maybe even more so.

LEARNING FROM NEGATIVE FEEDBACK

It was a whole new ballgame, all right. Some days, I seemed to be making progress; on others, it seemed as if I'd never really get the hang of it. One of the hardest lessons was learning to deal with negative reactions. Whenever anyone suggested that I could have done something differently, that there was a better way—whenever a thumb was turned even slightly downward—I felt devastated. What I needed more than anything was some honest feedback—what was working, what wasn't and how I could improve—but I found it excruciatingly difficult to accept.

I was hardly alone, according to Hal Johnson, managing director of Norman Broadbent International. "Men know that direct feedback isn't personal," he says, "but women are still learning this. They aren't used to having someone tell them directly that they screwed up. They don't know where this response is coming from—is it malicious or catty or jealous, or what?"

On his first day at a new job, Johnson recalls, the boss called him in and asked him what the hell he was doing wearing his pajama top. "Tweed sport jackets had been hot at my previous job," Johnson says with a chuckle. "How was I supposed to know that they were the kiss of death in New York?"

Although his boss came down on him like a ton of bricks, he says, he was actually doing him a big favor by keeping him from starting out on the wrong foot. Such in-your-face feedback often doesn't feel that great even to men, Johnson says, but not getting it is worse. "A guy learns he's in hot water right away," he says. "All too often, a woman doesn't know until it's too late."

Sometimes, even when you find out what the real score is, you still don't fit in. And such was the case for me and XYZ. I had felt like a failure—and a resentful one at that—until I actually sat down and scoped out the situation. Eventually, with much reflection and a lot of internal stock-taking, I could see that to get ahead I would have to adjust my style to theirs; I'd have to fit in. It did not seem unreasonable or impossible. But I could also see that I didn't want to do it. I had my own agenda, and I wanted to stick to it.

Once you've decided to leave, the next step is to figure out how to use your current job to help you move on. In my own case, I wanted to write full-time. From my experience at XYZ, I knew the topics that would be of interest there. So presto! I proposed a contract writing about those topics. Shortly afterward, contract under my arm, I took off. More important, I took off feeling good about myself. And I took off feeling good about those who stayed. XYZ wasn't right for me, but it was for them, and now I knew why.

—Gwenda Blair

HELLO, THIS IS YOUR DESTINY CALLING

WHETHER IT'S CATERING OR WRITING, SEWING CUSTOM DRAPES OR OPENING A BOUTIQUE, YOU MIGHT FIND YOUR HEART'S DESIRE IF YOU REALLY FOLLOW YOUR DREAMS.

I have a friend named Martha who had a dream during her second year of law school. She dreamed that she was a judge (an ambition her father always had for his only child) presiding over a courtroom. Martha sat, gavel in hand, listening to an attorney drone on and on. Suddenly in her dream Martha saw herself raising the gavel, which transformed into a dripping paintbrush. After her dream, she realized she could no longer ignore her desire to paint.

Martha, now an established visual artist, left law school, to her father's chagrin, and she has never looked back. While she was busy pursuing the career others had in mind for her, her dreams led her to her true calling.

There is a difference between a job, a career and a calling. What interests me the most is the calling. A calling, to me, is what our inner directives and creativity tell us we want to do with our lives, while a career—which may or may not also be a calling (I know many lawyers who long to

ON THE JOB

write novels)—usually provides us with an income in a respected profession such as medicine or newspaper editing. And a job is what we do to pay the bills, possibly while we are in pursuit of our calling, or simply to survive.

The artist who teaches, the cellist who works at my copy center—these individuals have taken jobs while they work at realizing their callings. It seems an odd quirk of life that often the things you love to do most are the things that are the least commercially viable.

But for those of us who have not yet discovered or who only have a vague sense of what our calling might be, it can take a long time to uncover what we really want to do (as well as what we are meant to do).

HEARING THE CALL

It took me years to realize that I was meant to be a writer. When I was a senior in high school, I wrote a poem, my first, and read it to my best friend in the back of English class one day. She listened to me and after a brief, awkward silence said she liked it. Of course, she was only being polite, because it was not a good poem, but I knew that I loved writing it.

It was as if everything I wanted to do and be had somehow swelled up inside of me into that startling moment when I put feelings into words and words onto paper. All I had ever felt—grief, love, anguish, loss, adolescent turmoil—was suddenly made clear in the swirl of writing that poem.

Then I went off to college, where I majored at various times in biology, French literature, musicology, archaeology and premed. I spent a tedious summer splaying dogfish and carving formaldehyde-soaked cats in a lugubrious laboratory, which would be the end of my medical career.

After college I toyed with this job and that, asking myself if there was something I loved to do. And I remembered that I had loved writing that poem. Of course I had been writing over the years, but it never occurred to me that this was something I could seriously pursue. Still I knew that I felt the most at peace, the most focused, when I was writing.

I went to my father and asked if he could help me for a year. I had worked it all out on paper. With some savings, my earnings from a part-time teaching job that wasn't terribly demanding and a small loan from my family, I could take a year to see if I could be a writer. My father said, "Just because you can toss a football doesn't mean you're going to be the quarterback."

"Well, I think I can do this," I said, meaning that I wanted to do this.

I was lucky. Many women (as well as men) over the years have struggled with economic and societal constraints, parental or spousal expectations or the demands of children that stand in the way of one's calling. But I was fortunate in that I not only recognized what I wanted, I also found the means and support to try to achieve my goal.

QUESTING FOR THE FUTURE

In Native American cultures, discovering one's calling is an important part of coming of age. The Lakota Sioux, for instance, encourage their adolescents to embark upon what they call "the vision quest." For young males, especially, the vision quest is a ritual that helps them define what direction their lives should take. After purifying oneself through sweating and depriving oneself of food, water and sleep, the vision may come as a dream, a sign, a spoken word. It may be brought by a messenger such as a deer or a crow. Once the vision is interpreted, the young person knows the direction of his or her life.

Not all of us have a mountaintop retreat where we can go to envision the course we should take toward creative self-fulfillment. But what Native American culture shows us is that we might, at some point, want to take time out and walk along a similar solitary road toward self-discovery. But how does one begin?

A key to one's personal question is this: to find what you want to do you must first learn to recognize your *own* uniqueness. In his autobiography, Pablo Casals, the renowned cellist, writes that we should say to our children, and to ourselves, "Do you know what you are? You are a marvel. You are unique. You may become a Shakespeare, a Michelangelo, a Beethoven. You have the capacity for anything. . . ."

Recognizing your uniqueness means paying attention to what it is that interests you. If you liked to be told stories as a child, you might like to write them or help publish them as an adult. If you liked to play tennis and race around, you might want to pursue a life's work that has to do with physical activity. Whether you like to look at images in *Life* magazine or correct people's grammar or help plants grow, look closely at where your interests lie and what makes you feel satisfied. Then use the answers to these questions as a clue to direct you toward what you want to do.

One of the best ways to clear your path toward recognizing your calling is to try to get rid of the "shoulds" and "cans." "I should earn $60,000 a year." "I can sew beautiful dresses, so I should sew them." But what if you earned less and were more fulfilled? What if, even though you can sew, you don't really like it?

I have a friend who became a doctor. It was what she thought she wanted to do, and she was good at it. Medicine was also a good way for her to earn a living. But my friend didn't like working with people's bodies. She used to tell me about it. "I don't like to touch then," she would say, chagrined. "I like to talk to them."

She didn't like surgical procedures or blood, but she liked to hear the patients talk about how they were feeling. After years of struggling with this, she did a residency in psychiatry (at great cost in both time and money to her family). Now she is a successful counselor, dealing specifically with the chronically ill.

FACING YOUR FEARS

Pursuing what you want to do and achieving your goal is not like finding the burning bush or discovering a gold mine. There are usually no epiphanies, no sudden reversals of fortune. Fulfillment comes in fits and starts. At its best, the decision to pursue what interests us can be a terrifying one, fraught with insecurity and doubt (in my experience, however, the people best at what they do are often fraught with insecurity and doubt). And there is, more often than not, tremendous risk involved.

The risk and uncertainty that come with our calling become apparent when reading the journals of renowned writers such as Gustave Flaubert and John Steinbeck, or the photographer Edward Weston. These were not people who got up each day and said, "I'm so talented, look at me," and breezed through work and life. Rather, they accepted each workday as a struggle and a challenge, often with a sense that their efforts might fail. In his journal to *Grapes of Wrath*, for instance, Steinbeck writes: "I'm afraid this book is going to pieces. If it does, I do too." It is not that you wake up one morning and say, "This is it," or "I can do this." Rather, it is as if every day you begin again.

People are always saying to me, "Oh, you're so lucky. You're a writer. You can work anywhere. You make your own hours." I also pay my own health insurance. I have no job security, and my hours are about the same as my tailor down the street who works at all hours. And we both get paid by the piece.

The fact is that I am a writer not because of the perks but because it is what I can do best. I've tried other things, and I can't do them. I decide to do something and on my way to doing it, I start to write again. As a friend once said, and this may be a good way to define a calling: While I was choosing it, it was choosing me.

Of course, I was very fortunate. Many circumstances could have kept me from having my chance. If my parents had sacrificed and struggled to send me through a premed program at an Ivy League college, I might have felt too much obligation and pressure to turn around later and say, "I want to write stories." For me, discovering and pursuing my life's calling didn't seem as impossible a task as it does for many.

Others are lucky because their dreams involve earning a

substantial amount of money, such as becoming a doctor or a lawyer. But often this is not the case. Learning how to follow our dreams is difficult if we don't feel we have a safety net. It is important to try to take the risk, and it is important to know that something or someone is there to catch you if you fall.

PROTECTING YOURSELF

Most writers and artists I know teach until they are absolutely sure they can make what is at best an unsteady income. Whether you are going off on a business venture on your own, tying up your capital in a restaurant or a store or taking a year off to see the world or paint landscapes, be sure to have something (preferably money) waiting for you when you return. Most creative or adventurous people I know are not foolhardy. There is nothing romantic about putting all your eggs in one basket.

For women, however, there are often not only financial risks and sacrifices but also emotional ones. In college when I read the biographies of women writers I admired such as Virginia Woolf, the Brontes and George Eliot, I was not surprised to learn that all were childless and few had what might be called a traditional marriage. It became obvious to me that, for the most part, the serious woman was the one who was willing to make a great personal sacrifice in terms of her family life.

Women, because of the needs of those they care for, have often had to defer their dreams. The writer Tillie Olsen has written eloquently about how the demands of domesticity, children and home have often kept women's voices silent. And Fay Weldon, when asked why she wrote shorter sentences in her early work, replied that when her children got older there was more time between interruptions.

By the same token, I once asked a well-respected American photographer—a man whose pictures hang in the finest museums—how he managed to do his art and raise three children. And he said somewhat absently, "Oh, it wasn't that difficult. Of course, my wife did most of the work."

OVERCOMING THE OBSTACLES

So how can we find a way in our life to do what Weldon did: adjust to her circumstances of raising children yet stay true to her vision? As the bills pile up (especially during a recession) and as our parents get older and the financial demands on us increase, how do we stay on course and be true to our calling?

In times of crisis like these we need to learn to pace ourselves. To write "shorter sentences," if you will. To adjust our vision to what is feasible for us to do at the time. Sometimes we are working, even if it is only in our head, while we are folding the laundry. Often, when it seems as if we are getting nowhere, we really are moving ahead.

The expectations we set for ourselves are the greatest curse. The Buddhists know this. That is why they put the focus on process—not on what you or others think you should be doing but rather on the simple task of breathing deeply and taking one step at a time. One foot in front of the other.

Often, even though we know what it is we want to do, there are real blocks to our fulfilling our dreams. The demands in our lives can be excessive. We think about the mortgage and put off our dreams for another day. And sometimes, if too much time has passed, it can feel as if it is too late for us. Yet while there are no guarantees, if you do the thing that you are really best suited for, chances are that eventually the world will recognize your efforts. If you do what you love, the money has been known to follow.

In many cases there are very real problems that stand in a woman's way. There are also women who have worked out their lives so that they are relatively free of the constraints of motherhood and earning a daily living yet find they are still unable to realize a life's dream. The mother of a friend lives on a large farm in upstate New York with perhaps a dozen solid structures on it. This woman longs to paint, yet she says she cannot find the room.

Excuses can get in the way. Lying to ourselves is a major pitfall. In the parable of the talents, Jesus says that the greatest sin of all is not using your God-given talent. And yet

many of us do not. Nothing seems more wasteful than someone who has something she wants to do in the world and is
stifled, not by circumstances but by herself.

GETTING OUT OF YOUR OWN WAY

This is the one obstacle when all others have been
removed that stands in our way. It is the most difficult
because it is not external—economic or social or even famil-
ial. Rather it comes from our internal lack of self-confidence:
the fear of failure, of taking a risk. Life is filled with ways we
can defeat ourselves. We wake up and say, "I want to write
like Faulkner or not write at all"; "I want to be Monet,
Truffaut, Madame Curie," and so on. We set our hopes too
high, and inevitably we fail.

Part of doing what we want means letting go of what we
don't do well. For instance, I long to be a runner, to run in a
marathon. Then I watch my husband sprint like a gazelle
around Prospect Park in Brooklyn and I have to admit that I
am a good walker, a glider on ice, a swimmer. But a runner, no.

Fulfillment comes in many guises, and it can come to us
in our lives at any time. But only we can make sure we will
be fulfilled. If we feel empty, no amount of water can fill our
well. It has to come from within, from the underground
springs and streams.

Personally, I don't think it matters what you do (unless
you are hurting people and/or committing a crime), as long
as it is what you want to do rather than fulfilling somebody
else's expectations of what you should be doing.

What is important isn't perfection; it's *possibility*. The
potential for doing good work, for making a film, for raising
a family, for being a good athlete. Let me suggest a simple
formula: possibility plus hard work plus a good dose of self-
confidence.

Know thyself, Socrates wrote. This is the hardest lesson
of all. To know what we really love. What we should hold
on to, what needs letting go of. Know what your gifts are,
then how to use them. And how do you know if you love to
do something? Because it will feel good when you do it.

Because the din of the world will go away and all your attention will be focused right there, on the thing you are doing. Watch a child who has found something she loves to do. It is all quite obvious to her.

—*Mary Morris*

SCORING A RAISE

GONE ARE THE DAYS WHEN YOU COULD EXPECT AN AUTOMATIC PAY INCREASE. IN THE 1990S, EARNING MORE BUCKS OR PERKS TAKES A LITTLE TALENT AND A LOT OF TACT.

From IBM and Sears to Ruby's Corner Store, downsizing and layoffs are the facts of life nowadays. As a result, you may be shouldering more responsibility without seeing any extra compensation. Should you be happy to have a job at all and forget about money? No way. Scoring a raise may be tougher than usual, but it's still possible.

Or maybe your job is safe—but structured so you can't ask for a raise and instead are handed a predetermined amount once a year. Does that mean you're stuck? Not necessarily. There are routes to working out a better deal, in money or perks.

Time it right. Bad timing when asking for a raise is like bad timing on a date—it can blow your chances. If your firm just announced massive layoffs or lost an important client, it's not a great time to try. On the other hand, if two years have gone by without so much as a cost-of-living dime thrown into your check, it's high time to request a raise. And, says Ginny Stratson, a chemist in Houston, Texas, "It never hurts to ask for more money when management is in love with you." She asked for—and got—a pay increase a week after her research project was written up in a major journal of science.

Take on more. You're expected to do a good job. Now shift into overdrive and take on more. Says David Cox, a former manager at IBM, "Nothing impressed me more than an employee who came to me with a written set of objectives that went above and beyond her job description. She said, 'If I accomplish this list, I'd like to discuss a raise.' She did everything on the list and got her increase."

Taking on more responsibility may mean doing some grunge work. Rose Lindsay, a nurse in Los Angeles, volunteered to work Saturday nights, since this was a tough slot for her boss to fill. "Sure, I hated working weekends. My social life was zilch, and I never slept," she says. "But management really appreciated my effort. Soon I got better assignments, which led to a promotion—without weekend work—and more money."

Brag a little. "Your boss doesn't care if you bought a house, had a baby or need new clothes," says Susan Kleinman, author of *Real Life 101: The Graduate's Guide to Survival.* "Raises are a reward for accomplishments. What have you done to help the company make money or do things better?" Keep records of your sales increases, productivity, creative projects and letters of goodwill from customers. Present them in writing. Don't worry if this seems immodest. Women are taught not to brag, but to negotiate a raise, you must toot your own horn.

Meet with your boss. Don't simply bop in, plop down in a chair and say, "Got a minute to talk dough-re-mi?" Make a formal appointment. Don't be late for it. And dress nicely. Look your boss in the eye. Keep your emotions in check, but don't be a robot either. Be assertive—not belligerent, but no sniveling either. The points you discuss should be well thought out and complete. Make sure you have answers to all possible responses.

Do your homework. Two tricky areas. *One:* the token increase. If you make $30,000, 2 percent a year is $600—that comes to a big $11.53 a week before taxes. Don't spend it all in once place. Work out the numbers before going to your boss. In 1991, raises averaged between 6.1 and 6.5 percent, and in 1992, between 4.5 and 4.7 percent.

Two: If more money is out of the question, suggest other forms of compensation, such as flextime, time off, job training, tuition reimbursement or maybe extra insurance benefits. "Paying for courses shows the company is investing in you, which will probably lead to a raise down the road," Kleinman explains.

Talk to co-workers. The recession is supposedly over, but its effects will be with us for years. Some bosses will use the economy as an excuse to save money for as long as possible. How do you know whether it's legitimate or just a dodge? Check with others at your company to see if they've received raises—chances are, they'll leak some information. "Some will talk about percentage increases, some won't, but they'll usually say if their pay went up," observes *Newsweek* money columnist Jane Bryant Quinn. Don't go in to your boss and whine: "No fair. Jennifer got a raise and I didn't." But let it be known you're aware the company is rewarding people.

Face the sad facts. If your boss says no anyway, take a deep breath and say, "Could we discuss this again in three months?" Period. Don't pick a fight, argue, dig in your heels or threaten to quit. The sad fact is that no one is indispensable. "Quitting when refused a raise is childish," says Melody Sharp Quarnstrom, author of *Getting on Top.*

"Despite all your good work, the only thing that will be remembered is your tantrum. And you need the boss for a reference." If you're mad enough to quit, keep it to yourself, but get to work on your résumé. If you quit before finding another job, you'll be in a financial hole in six months.

Don't quit, unless . . . "Never threaten to quit unless you have another job lined up," advises Marilyn Moats Kennedy, author of *Office Warfare.* But let's say you do have another offer—giving your boss a chance to match it might be a dangerous strategy. "Your boss may keep you for the moment but replace you when it's more convenient," says Kennedy.

A boss who insists that a raise is not in your future is sending you a message. "Take this seriously," says Kennedy. You probably should be looking for another job.

—*Cindy Pearlman*

HOW TO GET
A BETTER-PAYING JOB

TIRED OF WORKING ROUND THE CLOCK WITH STILL NO RAISE IN SIGHT? HERE ARE PROVEN STRATEGIES FOR DOUBLING YOUR SALARY IN FIVE YEARS.

Want to increase your income but don't know how? Consider the case of Mary Beth Sullivan, 42, now a successful stockbroker in New York City. Sullivan is living proof that a can-do attitude and a bit of hard work will bring quick salary advancement.

Sullivan, who has her master's degree in education, was teaching business courses at Burlington County College in New Jersey in the early 1980s when she realized that teaching had become humdrum. "There just wasn't room for creativity in my job," she says. There wasn't room for advancement or pay raises, either: after eight years, Sullivan was making about $17,000 a year.

What interested her more than her teaching duties was her modest investment account, which she traded herself. "I called up an old friend who was a stockbroker and asked him for advice on how to get into the brokerage business," she recalls. After interviewing at several firms, Sullivan joined the New York City—based investment firm of Smith Barney as an account executive trainee and toiled days and some evenings establishing an impressive client roster. In less than five years, she had more than doubled her salary; now, after ten years, she is a vice president at the firm. She made about $90,000 in 1991.

More and more women like Sullivan are willing to take risks to get out of dead-end jobs with paychecks that are on permanent hold. What are they realizing? That great careers don't simply fall into people's laps—they're pursued by job hunters in the 1990s as assiduously as prospectors panned for gold in the 1890s.

KNOWING WHEN TO MOVE ON

Do keep in mind that you can't move from job to job too often. Rita Calvo, president of Caliber Personnel Agency in New York City, advises that early on in your career you stay on the job at least 18 months. Later, a stay of 2½ years is preferred. "Companies love to see stability. If you've jumped around a lot, people think there's a negative reason," she says.

Any change is risky, and job shifts are no exception. But with planning and preparation, you can make the right move. How to start on your salary-doubling path? Consider one of the strategies below; they're time-honored and proven ways to increase your pay.

SAME FIELD . . . DIFFERENT FIRM

So you've tried everything you can think of to advance yourself in your company and you're still at square one? It may be time to jump ship. Working women are learning what working men have known for years: rare is the person who ascends quickly—in both status and pay—within the very organization where she began her career. By sticking around at the same old salary, in fact, you may be losing buying power. Thanks to inflation, your dollar bought about 5 percent less in 1991 than in 1990. If you receive 5 percent yearly raises, you're only treading water.

Job counselors agree that the easiest way to increase your earnings is to change companies but remain in the same career field. "In a good economic climate, most people can command more money from a prospective employer than from their current one," says Calvo. A 15 percent increase is typical and not unreasonable to ask for when you move. If you switch companies for a 15 percent increase and then ask for annual raises of 10 percent, you will just about double your salary in five years.

If the economic climate is lousy, it may be wise to stay put in your job where you're a known and trusted quantity. But that doesn't mean forever. Most economic downturns, though unsettling, are fleeting—the average recession lasts less than 12 months, according to economists. Use the waiting time to map out your strategy.

To test the waters, call a few employment agencies or headhunters for interviews. Take along an updated résumé and lots of questions about where job growth is and how you might be able to position yourself with your existing skills to tap that growth.

Check your Sunday newspapers for names of agencies that you can call. As you'll see by the job openings these firms are advertising, some specialize in certain fields—such as computing, health care or law. Approach those agencies that seem to be strongest in your area of interest. But don't turn your life over to a recruiter and don't hesitate to reject any jobs that don't feel right to you.

NOW FOR SOMETHING DIFFERENT

Think it's time to pursue that alternate dream career? Join the growing ranks of people who are choosing to change their careers. According to Carole Hyatt, author of *Shifting Gears*, 12 million people are currently engaged in switching to a new career, and 12 million more are actively planning the change. Indeed, trends indicate that the average person will have three distinct careers in her working life, says Hyatt.

One of the most successful ways to boost your salary in five years is to switch to a lucrative career field like sales, as stockbroker Sullivan did. You can also boost your salary by changing to a field that is related to your current one but pays more. For instance, a switch from commercial publishing to medical publishing or corporate communications will typically increase your salary, as will a switch from catalog copywriting to advertising copywriting.

Making the dramatic switch to a new career can seem daunting, especially if you're not sure what you would like to be doing. Begin by making a list of industries that interest you and why. Then do a little soul-searching: list your skills and what you love and loathe about your current and any recent jobs. What motivates you in your work? What do you daydream about doing? What were your favorite courses in college and why?

When casting about for a new career that will suit you, start by identifying preferences that will ensure your job satisfaction. According to *The Women's Job Search Handbook*, by Gerri Bloomberg and Margaret Holden, you must clarify three different issues—content, condition and compensation, the "three Cs."

Content addresses the question of what you want to do on a daily basis—what work will appeal to you and keep you challenged. Condition refers to the size and type of organization you would like to work for as well as its location, benefits and environment. And compensation: How much do you need to earn, not only to make ends meet but also to keep your self-esteem high?

Job counselors can help you find a rewarding new career. These professionals will tell you which industries are likely to be hot in coming years—such as the health-care or biotechnology fields—advise you on how to open doors in these industries and administer tests that will help identify your strengths and skills. Look for these advisers in the telephone book under Vocational Guidance or Counseling Services.

How do you sell yourself in a new industry? First, figure out what your transferable skills are. Having skills that are applicable to the new field is key to a successful switch. By angling your résumé and cover letter to highlight these talents, you'll help convince potential employers that you can do the job, even if you don't have solid experience in their industry.

Next, do your homework. Go to a local library or a nearby university library to investigate the industry you've targeted and the company you're seeing. Among the many business-related books and directories you might consult are *The Directory of Corporate Affiliations* (published by National Register Publishing Company in Wilmette, Illinois), an overview of about 4,000 major U.S. companies and their approximately 40,000 subsidiaries and affiliates; *Directory of Executive Recruiters* (published by Kennedy Publications in Fitzwilliam, New Hampshire), which lists over 2,000 recruiters in the United States, Canada and Mexico; and *Dun's Employment Opportunities Directory* (published by Dun's Marketing Services in Parsippany, New Jersey), which describes career opportunities and hiring practices of 5,000 U.S. companies.

Armed with facts about both the industry and the company you're seeing, you'll be better able to persuade your interviewer that you can address his or her immediate needs. This is crucial. According to David Bowman and Ronald Kweskin in their book *How Do I Find the Right Job? Ask the Experts*, your interview is your only chance to show what you can bring to the prospective employer's party. "Tell the interviewer how you can (1) help solve a department's problems, (2) bring new ideas to the company, (3) reduce costs and (4) increase sales or profits."

How you present yourself during the interview is important, too. In a survey conducted by Frank S. Endicott, former director of placement at Northwestern University, the following are the top five reasons employers gave for rejecting a job candidate: poor personal appearance, overbearing attitude, inability to express self clearly, lack of planning for career (no goals) and finally, lack of confidence and poise.

It all boils down to marketing yourself. In *The Job Hunt*, author Robert B. Nelson lists nine selling points that many job hunters have but overlook. These include: a broad and fresh perspective on the job; the ability to solve problems and think critically; a "learning" attitude and ability to adapt to change; energy, enthusiasm, motivation, initiative; and low cost compared with more experienced candidates.

TRY DOWNSIZING

The security of holding a job in a large U.S. corporation used to have great appeal to working women. But with all of the big-firm layoffs taking place today, job security is no longer guaranteed at even the most established companies.

Perhaps realizing this, many job-hoppers are finding that small firms—those with 500 employees or less and no more than $50 million in annual sales—are the place to go for both career and salary advancement. According to James Challenger, president of the Chicago-based outplacement firm Challenger, Gray and Christmas, employees find increased job satisfaction—more challenges, responsibility, feedback and opportunities—in smaller companies. They also make more money.

"Because smaller firms aren't able to get the talent that big firms can, they're willing to pay more," says Challenger. Big firms are more prestigious and viewed (again, not always correctly) as more secure places to work, so they are targeted by more job hunters.

A small company that's growing fast will typically look to the staffs of large companies for recruits. Jude Rich, chairperson of Sibson and Company, a management consulting firm in Princeton, New Jersey, explains what often happens: A small firm might pluck a junior employee from a large firm and give her a promotion and the additional money that the promotion involves.

"Moving up to a bigger job can mean a 20 percent to 40 percent increase in salary," he says. Although this isn't happening in all industries, especially during today's economic slowdown, such increases are being paid to recruits in marketing, finance and manufacturing jobs. The practice is especially prevalent in the consumer-products business.

Of course, there are downsides to moving to a smaller firm. Often these companies are located off the beaten path, in small towns or exurban areas where expenses are lower than they are in big cities. Moving to one of these companies may require that you do your starting over in a brand-new town, a frightening prospect to even the most adventuresome. But if, unlike many job applicants, you're willing to move, you may find yourself landing the job of your dreams.

SEARCH OUT THE SMALL FRY

Don't want to move? Try hunting for jobs in small-town or suburban areas near your home. This might require that you do a reverse commute, but you could land a higher-paying job as a result. Consider one 33-year-old editor who recently switched from a magazine job in New York City to one in a nearby suburb. The new job did require a reverse commute, but it also raised her salary significantly—by 30 percent.

One source of information on more obscure employers is newspaper classified ads. If you know an area you might like to move to, get a copy of the largest Sunday paper that serves that locale and comb through the want ads. If you're unsure of where you would be inclined to move, consult the *Wall Street Journal*. It carries ads from employers around the nation.

Another way to target smaller firms is to look at companies that are customers of the company you are currently working in, or conversely, make a list of those firms that are your company's suppliers. If you work at a cosmetics company, for example, consider both your suppliers—chemical, packaging and equipment vendors—and your customers—distributors and retailers. Both are apt to be smaller concerns that speak your language and know you from your company.

Making a move—whether across town or across country—takes courage and action. But success rarely comes to those who sit still. As Lee Iacocca, former chairman of Chrysler Corporation, once said: "The trick is to make sure you don't die waiting for prosperity to come."

—*Gretchen Morgenson*

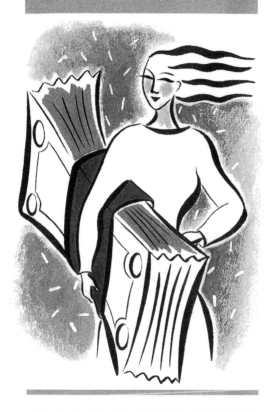

PART SIX

MANAGING YOUR MONEY

IT PAYS TO COMPLAIN

AN EFFECTIVE COMPLAINT LETTER CAN PRODUCE
SURPRISING RESULTS—REPLACEMENTS, REFUNDS,
GIFT CERTIFICATES, FREE SAMPLES, EVEN IMPROVED
PRODUCTS AND SERVICES.

It was a day to forget. First, I noticed that the band on my six-month-old watch was coming apart. (The safety chain had broken already.) Then the boy behind the fast-food counter was rude to me. Finally, my health insurance company rejected $790 in claims that I submitted.

Was I depressed? Yes. Was I angry? Absolutely. How could I get rid of those feelings? I decided to retaliate. I sat down and typed three complaint letters to the companies in question.

Within four weeks, my watch sported a new band and safety chain, even though they were not covered by the warranty. Representatives from the fast-food restaurant called me twice and sent a letter of apology, including two coupons for free food. And the insurance company reexamined my claims and agreed to pay 90 percent of the bills.

In the past five months, I've written more than 25 complaint letters to companies ranging from manufacturers of toys and medical supplies to clothing suppliers. My response rate is 92 percent. I've received food coupons worth $16.50, $55 in gift certificates, products worth $98 and medical supplies valued at $149. I should have started my retaliation campaign sooner!

LETTERS GET THE MOST ACTION

As a remedial-writing instructor, I taught my students how to write effective complaint letters. The results of those they mailed were encouraging, but I never practiced what I preached. Instead, I fretted over flawed socks, badgered my husband to fix the broken stroller and swore I'd never return to a restaurant whose employees gave me poor service.

My husband grew tired of my complaints and urged me to write letters instead. I did and quickly learned the emotional and financial rewards of effective complaints. Suddenly, I was in control. And in helping myself, I felt I was helping to improve products and services for others. When I complained about a split seam in an infant coverall, for example, the company promised to increase seam allowances and reinforcements.

You also can reap the rewards of effective complaint letters by following these steps.

Be sure your complaint is valid. Don't approach a company with a problem that's your own fault or stems from a misunderstanding. Make sure you have followed directions and have been reasonable in your expectations.

Save all parts and relevant papers. It helps to have the model or serial number, warranty and receipt when you write to complain. Never throw away the broken product; the company may ask to examine it. I used to discard receipts after I'd worn a garment once or used a small appliance a few times without mishap. Now I know it pays to save them.

Type your letter. A neatly typed letter makes a better impression than a handwritten one and improves your chances of a good response. Always check it for errors before mailing.

Address your letter correctly. Most companies list their address on the packaging, the warranty card and instruction booklets. If you need the corporate headquarters, consult *Standard & Poor's Register of Corporations, Directors and Executives* in the library. Call a store or restaurant for the address of their corporate headquarters. Most stores also can supply addresses of manufacturers of the products they carry.

Write to the person in charge. And be sure to get the correct spelling of his or her name from *Standard & Poor's Register* or by calling the firm's 800 number.

You needn't write the president of the company over a

small matter. Someone at a lower level may provide better and faster results—especially if you send a copy to the president and indicate that at the bottom of the letter. When a box of my favorite crackers were undercooked, I received prompt results from the customer-service manager. But when the safety of my children was at risk because of an unsafe toy, I went straight to the top.

Establish rapport in your opening. The person who receives your letter will be more eager to help if you're a loyal customer and say so. If you've never purchased their products or patronized their store before, explain why you did so this time. Learning that you love the firm's advertising or admire its reputation for top quality puts the recipient of your letter in a positive frame of mind.

State the problem succinctly. A few paragraphs are usually sufficient to explain your complaint. Include a careful description of the product, the model or serial number and copies of relevant papers. If your problem relates to service, include relevant dates, times, locations and names of employees, when possible.

Don't write when you're angry. Wait until you've calmed down, then write on the assumption that the recipient of your letter cares about your problem and is eager to help you resolve it.

Ask for a specific resolution in clear-cut cases only. When my son's stroller snapped going over a curb and couldn't be fixed, I requested a replacement. But I'm glad I didn't request a replacement when I complained about a pair of flawed socks. I received two pairs of better-quality socks in return! Specific requests may limit your chances of a more generous settlement.

End on a positive note. Write that you hope the problem can be resolved quickly so that your confidence in the company will be restored. A thank-you for assistance is always appreciated. Include your phone number in case the person wants more information.

Make a copy of your letter before mailing. If the company does not respond in four to six weeks, send a copy with a note expressing your disappointment at not receiving a response. If you didn't write the president the first time, send him or her the follow-up letter.

Don't give up. If you still don't get a response or you're not satisfied, contact the Better Business Bureau. For insurance problems, contact your state's insurance commissioner. If your complaint involves an unsafe product, write to the Consumer Product Safety Commission, Washington, DC 20207. A complaint about possible fraud should be addressed to your state's attorney general or, if mail is involved, to Charles R. Clauson, Chief Postal Inspector, U.S. Postal Inspection Service, 475 L'Enfant Plaza, S.W., Washington, DC 20260.

Send a thank-you letter to anyone who is extremely helpful. This courtesy should give the company incentive to continue helping customers.

—Ruth Nauss Stingley

BE YOUR OWN FINANCIAL PLANNER

IT DOESN'T PAY TO LET OTHERS MAKE ALL THOSE IMPORTANT DECISIONS ABOUT MONEY. HERE'S WHAT YOU NEED TO KNOW TO TAKE CHARGE OF YOUR OWN FINANCES.

Me, be my own planner? You must be kidding."

That's what I'd have said back in the days when the financial world was a mystery to me. On the advice of so-called experts, I even bought into an oil well that was dry and a company whose stock went down, down, down.

Half a lifetime later, I've learned that the best financial

plans are simple—so simple you can run them yourself. You need only a well-defined list of goals and a few plain-vanilla financial products, plus a clear understanding of how each of them works.

Many women don't want to think about money. They turn to their husbands or fathers for advice, perpetuating their dependence. Or they hand everything over to financial planners, some of whom give terrible advice. A planner might even sell you a very risky investment just to earn the high sales commissions it pays.

To avoid losing money—or wasting it—you must become well informed about personal finance. Fortunately, basic money management is not difficult. The best source of current news and strategies is *Kiplinger's Personal Finance Magazine,* at $18 a year. The library has many personal-

WHEN TO SEE A PROFESSIONAL

Occasionally, you do need an expert opinion. An accountant or financial planner can help you with budgeting and long-term savings projections, for example. Consult a professional if:

• You earn good wages but cannot save a dime. You need to be shown, in dollars and cents, how poor you'll be at retirement if you don't start changing your habits now.

• Your questions can't be answered without technical expertise. If your employer offers early retirement alternatives, for example, you'll want to project how each might work out over your life expectancy.

• You wonder if an expert can improve your personal plan. Arrange for a meeting at an hourly fee. Accountants charge flat fees and usually sell no financial products. Most financial planners, however, sell insurance and/or mutual funds as well as advice. Make no decisions about changing your plan until you've gone home and thought it over very carefully.

finance books, such as my own latest, *Making the Most of Your Money*, and *The Fidelity Guide to Mutual Funds* by Mary Rowland.

Classes on money management and investing, often sponsored by senior citizen groups or community colleges, are widely available. But be wary of those taught by stockbrokers or financial planners. When teachers push products they sell, you're getting a sales pitch, not an education.

Here's how to create your own financial plan from the ground up.

Make a list of financial objectives. These will change over the years but might include:

- Get out of debt by doubling monthly credit card payments.
- Save $10,000 by 1996 for a down payment on a house.
- Accumulate $20,000 in ten years for college tuition.
- Save $1,000 for a vacation next year.
- Contribute 5 percent of every paycheck to a retirement savings plan.

Your own goals may be lower or higher, but whatever your objective, be specific. "Save money" is only a vague hope; "save $100 a month toward a $2,000 nest egg" is a goal you can reach. Each goal should be broken down into monthly sums you can check off.

Draw up a budget that meets your objectives. Start with a "baseline budget" that shows current spending. Go through old checkbooks to see what you spent in the last six months, then carry a notebook to record all your cash outlays for the next month. List them under budget headings—

WHEN NOT TO SEE A PROFESSIONAL

Don't consult a financial planner who earns a living selling mutual funds and other financial products unless you are knowledgeable about personal finance. Without such knowledge, you won't be able to judge whether the advice you're getting is good or downright disastrous.

---

groceries, transportation, telephone, clothing, lunch.

Next, work out an ideal budget that puts your specific goals at the top. For example, the top line might read "$200 more a month toward credit card debt." That $200 is then put aside every month, before you spend on anything else. Divide what's left among the other categories. Be sure to establish a reserve fund for unpredictable expenses, such as veterinary bills or appliance repairs.

Make a third budget column labeled "actual." Enter your expenditures weekly. At the end of each month, compare your ideal plan with what you really spent. If you're spending more than you intended on "telephone" or "clothing," you may have to strengthen your resolve—or adjust your goals. After several months, you should arrive at a reasonable budget you can live with.

Have faith that you can save. You might think it's impossible, but you could put 5 percent of every paycheck into the bank without nicking your standard of living. I know, because I tried it at age 27 when I thought I hadn't a penny extra—and managed to capture money that was slipping through my fingers. Since then, I've seen automatic 5 percent savings plans work for hundreds of other people. One more tip: Before putting this money into your savings account, use it to reduce your debt. The less interest, the more money you'll have to spend or save.

Secure what you have. Buy inexpensive insurance to protect you and your family. Here are the most important things to know about each type.

Life insurance: A family of four needs coverage equal to seven times their annual income. If you earn 40 percent of the income, you should carry 40 percent of the insurance. Single people with no dependents don't need life insurance.

Auto insurance: The best way to cut the price is to shop around. Start with a price quote from State Farm, which sells through agents, and the Government Employees Insurance Company (750 Woodbury Rd., Woodbury, NY 11797), which sells by mail. Then ask an independent insurance agent if he or she can find you something cheaper.

Homeowners' insurance: You should be insured for 100 percent of the cost of rebuilding your home from the foundation up, in case of a total wipeout. Never let your coverage fall below 80 percent of rebuilding costs or you won't be reimbursed in full for lesser claims. Consider "replacement cost" coverage, even though the premiums are higher. Regular policies pay only what your furniture would be worth secondhand; replacement-cost policies give you enough money to buy new furniture.

Disability insurance: This pays you an income if you're unable to work, but it's affordable only to workers in white-collar occupations.

Health insurance: If you don't have coverage at work, check into group coverage through a union, trade association or health maintenance organization (HMO). If you have to buy an individual policy, the best way to lower your costs is to take a big deductible.

Create an investment plan. Here are the essentials you need to know about investment risk.

Stock-market investors face a real risk of loss over short periods, like one to four years. Money you'll need soon (such as your rainy-day fund, savings toward a down payment on a house or other major purchases and money your teenager will need for college within four years) should be kept absolutely safe and accessible. A rainy-day fund belongs in a money market mutual fund or a savings account in a federally insured bank. Short-term college savings can go into Series EE Savings Bonds (middle-income families pay no income tax on the interest when EE bonds are used for tuition).

Stock investments are hardly risky at all over periods of five years or more. If you buy good mutual funds and hold, through thick and thin, for at least five years, the odds are high that you'll come out way ahead. This is the place for retirement funds and college savings for young children. Since 1947, stocks have returned an average of 13.5 percent compounded annually.

For a directory of more than 100 mutual funds with no sales charges, send $3 to the 100% No-Load Mutual Fund Council, 1501 Broadway, Suite 1809, New York, NY 10036. You might ask leading no-load mutual fund groups to send you information about each of their funds. These groups include Scudder, Twentieth Century and Vanguard.

To make sure you invest regularly, arrange for money to be taken from your bank account automatically each month and put into mutual fund shares. For example, you might invest $50 a month in a bond fund paying a high current return and $100 a month in a stock fund that offers more growth potential. That way your investments build up without your thinking about them.

Set up a tax-deferred retirement savings plan. Your employer may offer one through a 401(k) or other payroll-deduction plan. Contribute as much as you can, especially if your company matches what you put in. That's like picking up gold in the streets. Since no taxes are withheld from contributions, they don't reduce your take-home pay as much as many people think.

Employees with no company plans should start Individual Retirement Accounts; the self-employed should start Keogh plans. The best place for both accounts is a good mutual fund group.

—Jane Bryant Quinn

SCRIMPING: WHEN IT PAYS OFF

SOMETIMES PINCHING THOSE PENNIES PAYS OFF IN WONDERFUL WAYS. AND SOMETIMES THE DEPRIVATION JUST ISN'T WORTH IT. HERE'S HOW TO TELL THE DIFFERENCE.

Vicki, who lives in a big city, would rather wait 20 minutes for a bus on a blustery day than spend $4 to hop a cab home. She brown-bags it for lunch, reads the office copy of the newspaper instead of buying her own, never orders an appetizer when she eats out and makes long-distance calls only after 11:00 P.M.

Is Vicki a miser? Not at all: Her economies have bought her a condominium apartment. After years of living with roommates, she decided two years ago to buy her own place, even though it was a big financial stretch.

"On my salary, a mortgage hasn't been easy," she says. "But precisely because I'm not in a high-paying field, I figured that if I wanted my own home I'd better jump while the market was in a slump. I wanted the privacy and independence, so for me this was the right decision."

Last spring, Kelly, a friend of Vicki's, decided to buy a top-of-the-line Camry with a cassette player, air conditioning and lots of other extras. The bill came to $20,000. Kelly had initially considered a $13,000, no-frills Chevrolet, but because she has a long commute to work, she decided she'd appreciate the more luxurious car. Her monthly payments on the Camry—which she'll be making for four years—are $392. The Chevy would have put her out only $240 a month. "For the first couple of months, I really enjoyed the car," says Kelly. "Then I got tired of worrying about what I was spending on clothes and even food. If I'd bought the Chevy, I'd have $150 a month more to spend on other things! How am I going to put up with this penny-pinching for three more years?"

LEARN THE RULES OF PENNY-PINCHING

At one time or another most of us want or need something that is slightly beyond our means—a vacation, a designer suit, tuition for graduate school—and getting it means scrimping. Sometimes we scrimp simply so that we can build savings for the future or for our retirement. But what is really worth scrimping for, and what's the best way to survive the deprivation? Here are a few guidelines.

Scrimp first, indulge later. It's easier to bear the pain of constant little economies when you're still reaching for the reward. Kelly's mistake was taking the reward—her new car—first. If it's not possible to follow this rule, make sure that you're getting something—an apartment, a graduate degree—that will continue to justify any ongoing belt-tightening.

Look for a fast payoff. The reward should not only come second, it should come quickly. You might not mind spending a few nights of your vacation in Spartan accommodations in order to dine at a world-famous restaurant on your final evening. On the other hand, eating tuna fish every day for three months before you even get on the plane could wear you down.

Determine your priorities. Vicki thought long and hard before buying her "too expensive" condo. Finally she decided: "I'm 30—I don't want to have to be married before I can feel settled. I knew the sense of permanence was going to be more important to me in the long run than financial flexibility. And things will get a little easier as I move up at my job."

Try to pinpoint what the thing you desire means to you—and what you'll have to give up to get it. Are you planning that expensive wedding because you want a big public celebration of an important day or because your sister had one? Even if it's the former, is it worth doing without decent furniture for the next three years to pay for the extravaganza? Only you can decide.

Don't get hung up on the small stuff. The lipstick you love because it's just the right shade and doesn't smudge off may cost $6 or $8 more than the brands you could buy at a discount drugstore. But you could spend twice that much testing $3 tubes to find one you can live with. When you've hit on a high-quality, reasonably durable product that's hard to duplicate, a few extra dollars amount to a good investment.

Remember that your time is also worth something. If you have a busy full-time job, the extra half hour per week you'll spend in the supermarket comparing prices on instant coffee and plastic wrap could probably be put to better use.

Certain items just aren't negotiable. If your office culture dictates a professional look at all times, forgoing a good haircut or a nicely tailored suit may cost you money—in raises and promotions.

Be aware that continual scrimping can take a toll on your personal relationships. Do you want to be known among your friends as the one who always insists on renting a video or eating at the local hole-in-the-wall when the others want to see a new movie or enjoy a leisurely dinner with a bottle of wine? When you notice your hardship tactics grating on other people's nerves, it's time to gracefully make an exception.

—*Barbara Gilder Quint*

RIPPED OFF! 19 WAYS TO PROTECT YOURSELF

BUYER, BEWARE. SOMETIMES IT SEEMS LIKE EVERYONE'S OUT TO GET YOU—FROM CON ARTISTS TO YOUR FRIENDLY SALESMAN. HERE'S HOW TO PROTECT YOURSELF.

Scams have been around for years—probably ever since there's been money—but in an economic downturn they really take root. "Con artists prey on the vulnerable," says Stephen Brobeck, executive director of the Consumer Federation of America. At risk: the down-and-out, the out-of-work, the overextended. But they're not alone. With get-rich-quick schemes also on the rise—from bogus home repairs to fraudulent car deals (even venerable Sears was caught overcharging for auto repairs)—the financially solvent are at risk, too.

The top trouble spots, according to the Consumer Federation of America: home repairs, mail-order sales, auto repairs and telemarketing scams. And as Al White, an investigative reporter for WWOR-TV in New York City, points out, there are plenty of perfectly legitimate practices that count on you not to read the fine print. So what's a consumer to do? Keep your wits about you, your pocketbook firmly closed—and educate yourself.

1. Store return policies. When you tried to return a toaster that scorched bread the first time you used it, the salesperson said all purchases were final. In truth, some purchases are less final than others. According to the National Uniform Commercial Code, you must be able to use a product for the purpose you bought it. If not, you're due a refund.

2. Easy loans. If a letter comes in the mail promising a fast loan—no questions asked—throw it right out. "If it sounds too good to be true, it probably is," says Anna Flores, executive director of the National Association of Consumer Agency Administrators in Washington, D.C. "Use your common sense: What credible lending institution would lend you money without making you qualify? The answer is, none."

3. Credit cards. One result of increased competition among banks: Credit card offers now flow your way, with promises of low rates, low fees, long grace periods. How can you weed out the hype? "Look for the lowest annual percentage rate or no annual fee," says Mary Beth Butler of the Bank Card Holders of America in Herndon, Virginia.

4. Mortgage payments. You're so in debt you're afraid you'll lose your house. Even so, don't believe any financial counselor who promises to postpone foreclosure if you give her a $500 fee up front, says Brobeck. If you're unfortunate enough to fall for this ruse, as some hapless Detroit residents did, you'll end up with nothing.

5. Unsolicited services. It's simple: "Never do business with anybody who knocks at your door. And always ask for references from any service people you plan to use," says William Young, director of consumer affairs for the National Association of Home Builders. If they're on the level, they should be able to produce a license or references. Demand estimates—in writing.

6. A diploma in no time. You need more training to get a better job, but you don't have much time or money. Before enrolling in a short-term vocational school, your best bet is to verify its accreditation with the Career College Association in Washington, D.C.

7. Genealogy books. What's in a name? For some folks, a lot of money. If you receive a postcard asking you to buy a history of your family, don't expect much. At best, what you'll get, according to Lorna Christie of the Direct Marketing Association, is just a volume that gives cursory definitions of hundreds of family names. Read the offer carefully.

8. Funeral costs. Looking for a good deal on a funeral? That may sound unseemly, but prices and services do differ significantly. The Federal Trade Commission, which regulates the funeral industry, requires every funeral home to disclose prices over the phone, says Robert J. Smith, president of the National Funeral Directors Association. "According to the law, the family must be given a printed general price list, itemizing expenses and explaining regulations."

9. Moving estimates. Ask for a binding estimate in writing, based on what's known as "constructive weight," advises Linda Mitchler, transportation industry analyst for the Interstate Commerce Commission. How is it established? Printed on the back of most moving contracts is a chart of standard weights for individual household items; those that apply in your case are added up to achieve your total. While you'll still have to pay for time lost due to such problems as unexpected stairs, you won't have to pay more for weight.

10. Phone calling cards. The key: Make sure no one can see you punch in your personal code. Memorize your number, advises Jim Snyder, special counsel for MCI Communications. Watch out for loiterers and stand directly in front of the phone, covering your hand while punching in the number.

11. Real estate. While house hunting, you've gotten to know your real estate agent well. She understands your financial situation and has your best interests at heart, right? Not necessarily, says Arthur Riolo, a real estate broker in Hastings-on-Hudson, New York. As he says, if the agent is working for the seller, she's just trying to seal the deal. And her guidance could cost you money—for example, she could encourage you to offer more than you really need to. That's why many states require real estate agents to provide potential buyers with disclosure statements that set out the ground rules and let all parties know who's really representing whom.

12. Telemarketing. Don't give out credit card numbers to anyone claiming he needs them for a marketing survey, advises Flores, or soon you may be billed for merchandise you never ordered. "Not all telemarketing companies are fraudulent," she explains. "Those that aren't will gladly give you their number and send you written material detailing their product."

13. Buying stocks. A stockbroker calls you and eagerly recommends a company that's about to launch a new product, with the stock's value sure to rise 25 percent. Before you write a check, think twice. "If an investment has the potential to go up 25 percent, it can also go down 25 percent—or more—in the same time," says Madeline I. Noveck, president of the Institute of Certified Financial Planners and president of Novos Planning Associates in New York City. The broker isn't purposely trying to mislead you, says Noveck; he's just trying to make the sale. It's up to you to ask the difficult questions. Ask for an analyst's report for more information, and take time to read everything you can about the company.

14. The advertised discount. You're in the market for a camera and you see one advertised below standard cost. When you stop by the store, the salesperson tells you the camera is out of stock. Besides, it won't meet your needs, he says, pulling out a more expensive model. Stick to your guns: This is a bait-and-switch scam. If you really want the cheaper item, ask for it. But be sure to ask if it comes with all its accessories—chances are the low price means there's a lot missing.

15. Getting your child into modeling. You receive a letter from an agency that promises to turn your child into a model. You go to the studio, only to find out there's a sizable up-front fee for the initial photo shoot. Before you sign up for overpriced photo sessions—which are how some agencies get around state laws deeming it illegal to charge a fee without providing a service—research the company to see if it's legit, says Clair Villano of the Denver district attorney's office.

16. Too good to be true. You see a mouth-watering ad for a resort vacation at a truly affordable price. You make your plans, send in your check, then find out your "plane tickets" are discount vouchers worth as little as $10 each; the accommodations are third-rate and the food is inedible. To prevent such a scenario, talk to a reputable travel agency or tour operator first, says Henry Herschel of the Missouri attorney general's office. Ask for names of people who have already taken the tour. And find out what's included in the package.

17. Buying jewelry. You find a diamond-studded gold brooch in a store that always seems to be running a sale. The weeks-old sale is your cue that this store may have marked up the jewelry by five or six times its value (even if it's now 50 percent off), says Elizabeth Lilly-Holbrook, a certified gemologist appraiser in West Virginia. (After all, how can any store stay in business very long if it's always running sales?) If the jewelry's on-sale price is $599 and the store claims its regular price is $799, you can bet its true value is the lower figure, says Lilly-Holbrook. Make sure you're dealing with a reputable dealer: Look for a store affiliated with the American Gem Society, which has a strict code of ethics.

18. Working at home. You see an ad promising you $500 a week for working at home: Just send $35 for a kit telling you how to make ornaments. "Before you send the money, stop and think. Why would you pay to work?" says

Villano. At best you'll probably receive only a useless instruction book.

19. Home repairs. You've hired someone to fix your air conditioner. Don't leave the house, says investigative reporter White. "Sometimes only a new fuse is added, but you'll be billed for more expensive repairs." White's advice: Stay put and ask questions.

—Michael Winkleman

LADY, IT'S GOING TO BE EXPENSIVE!

WHAT ARE THE ODDS OF YOUR BEING CHEATED BY AN AUTO MECHANIC? LET A MASTER MECHANIC TEACH YOU HOW TO AVOID RIP-OFFS.

Most people would rather have a root canal than take a car in for repairs. Whatever the problem—and let's face it, we usually have no idea what's wrong with the car—it's almost guaranteed to be expensive. And when it's time to pay that seemingly exorbitant bill, who really knows if all those new parts were necessary? Since few car owners truly understand what happens under the hood, especially with today's high-tech, computerized cars, many of us wonder if we've been the victim of a dishonest mechanic.

INVESTIGATING THE MECHANICS

To see just how honest service stations really are, Andrew Panagakos, a master technician certified by the National Institute for Automotive Service Excellence (ASE) and co-owner of the Texaco station in Maywood, New Jersey, taught me how to rig a 1990 Dodge Spirit to create two common repair problems. The first was a relatively simple and inexpensive problem: a nonworking headlight (we substituted a blown fuse for the good one).

The second malfunction was more ambiguous: With an injector wire partially unplugged, the car misfired on one cylinder and idled roughly, thus triggering the "check engine" light. Although time-consuming to locate, this problem requires no parts—the only charge should be for diagnostic time.

Before I began, the car was completely checked out by Panagakos, who has been repairing cars for over 16 years. He gave it a clean bill of health. Over the next three days, I chose two garages at random in each of three states. At half the stations, I had the headlight fixed; the other three dealt with the "check engine" light. To see whether my knowledge—or lack of knowledge—made any difference in how I was treated, I pretended to be very savvy about cars the first day, to have an average amount of knowledge the next day and to know absolutely nothing about cars on the third. Panagakos checked the repair work at the end of each day.

Here's what happened:

Day One: 10:15 A.M. My first stop was on Highway 46 in Clinton, New Jersey. I pulled into a parking lot just before I reached the station, checked my lights (both worked) and then substituted a blown fuse for the one that goes to the driver-side headlight. I checked again to be sure the headlight was out.

10:20 A.M. I drove to the station and told the mechanic my headlight was not working. While I watched, he replaced the bulb. Since the headlight still did not work, he put the old bulb back in and changed the fuse. Charge: $2 for the part, no charge for labor. Great! I had met an honest man.

11:00 A.M. The next station was in Cedar Grove, New Jersey. I partially unplugged the injector wire and drove into the station. Using the right lingo, I told the mechanic that my car was idling roughly, or missing, and that the "check engine" light was on. I said—with great authority—that I knew one cylinder was not firing and suspected a bad spark plug, spark plug wire or fuel injector (which was, in fact close to the truth, since the injector wire wasn't connected completely).

I also mentioned that the alternator belt had been changed recently, and it was possible that something had simply been knocked loose at that time. I told him the car had just had a tune-up three months ago. We went for a test drive, and the mechanic agreed that it was missing and that one of the possibilities I had mentioned was probably correct. I left the car with him and called every two hours to check on his progress.

5:05 P.M. Finally, I was told that the problem had been solved, and I went back to pick up the car. Total cost: $176.49 for a complete set of new spark plugs, new ignition wires, a new distributor cap and rotor, plus labor. So much for my authoritative stance! He said nothing about the loose injector wire. I asked to keep my old parts—they found everything but the rotor—and returned to Maywood.

5:20 P.M. I noticed on the way back that although the car was no longer missing, it was not running well.

6:15 P.M. I found out when I got back that not only did the Cedar Grove mechanic do a lot of unnecessary work, he did it badly. Panagakos discovered that the center electrode on my new distributor cap was broken, the mechanic hadn't fastened the air cleaner down after he changed the spark plugs and one of my new spark plug wires was cracked. I had been charged almost $200 for a slapdash job and defective parts. Panagakos reinstalled the original parts, which were still in good shape.

Day Two: 11:00 A.M. With the blown headlight fuse substituted, I stopped at a small garage in Suffern, New York. The mechanic, who couldn't have been a day over 19, quickly found that the bulb was fine, then tested and replaced the fuse. All for no charge. (He even checked the restroom for cleanliness when I asked to use it!)

1:10 P.M. I found the next station in Spring Valley, New York, and again I partially disconnected the injector wire. Since this was my day to act like I had an average amount of knowledge, I told the mechanic only that the car was obviously not running well and the "check engine" light was on.

I gave him basic information like the make and model of the car when he asked for it, but not much else. He did some initial checking while I waited and then came and told me that one cylinder was not firing. He drew a diagram of the engine to illustrate and kept repeating that the car was a six-cylinder. Apparently, what I thought was an average display of knowledge was interpreted by the mechanic as being just short of stupid. I left the car with him and called every hour or so until it was done.

5:35 P.M. When I picked up the car, he said, "I was able to locate the problem, and I repaired it." He didn't say what the problem was (and I didn't ask). He had also changed the spark plugs, he said, because the ones in the car were the wrong type. Out of curiosity, I did ask him to explain what he meant by "the wrong type." His answer was completely incomprehensible—perhaps because he was trying to avoid terms he thought I wouldn't understand—but it seemed to have something to do with the brand name of the spark plugs. The cost: $95.33 for computer diagnostic time and a new set of spark plugs.

6:45 P.M. Back at Panagakos' station, we found that the injector wire had indeed been found and plugged in. However, Panagakos discovered that the spark plugs in the car were the original ACs, not the Champions that the Spring Valley mechanic said he installed. Ripped off again! Wonder what he would have done if I had asked him to give me the old spark plugs?

Day Three: 12:15 P.M. This was my day to act dumb. In Cos Cob, Connecticut, I again installed the blown fuse, after checking the bulbs, and drove to the station. This time, after the mechanic agreed to check the headlight, I said I wanted to do some shopping at a store across the street and left the station.

12:35 P.M. When I returned, the attendant told me that he had changed my headlight bulb. The cost: $26.50. No mention of the fuse, although it had been replaced. Since we

(continued on page 174)

While a basic understanding of your car will not necessarily protect you from being cheated, it may decrease the odds. At the least, it should force a mechanic who does plan to cheat you to be much more careful, and perhaps you won't end up spending as much as you would have otherwise. One caveat: If you try to sound far more knowledgeable than you really are, you're likely to make a mistake and end up sounding foolish.

Here are a few things you can do to protect yourself from dishonest mechanics.

Read your owner's manual, cover to cover. This may sound like simplistic advice, but you'll be amazed at what you learn, even if you think you know a lot about your car. (If your car is old or used and the manual is missing, write to the manufacturer.)

Know the make and model of your car. And memorize your license plate number. (You'll usually be asked to fill out a form with this information, as well as your name, address and phone number.)

Know how many cylinders your car has. Also, know if it is a front-wheel, rear-wheel or four-wheel drive.

Know the location of the hood release inside the car and the latch under the hood itself. You should also know where to find the dipsticks for oil and transmission fluid and where to add windshield washer fluid, brake fluid and antifreeze.

Keep accurate records of regular maintenance and repairs. This information includes oil changes, tune-ups and new tires. You'll sound like a pro if you casually mention that the car just had a tune-up at 40,000 miles.

Pay attention to your gas mileage. Any sudden change can be an indication that something is wrong.

Getting the Most from Your Car

Here's what you need to know to extend the life of your car and cut down on repairs in the first place.

Have the car serviced regularly. You'll find

the recommended intervals for oil changes and tune-ups in your owner's manual. However, Andrew Panagakos, a master technician and co-owner of the Texaco station in Maywood, New Jersey, says that since most cars are driven harder than what is considered normal by manufacturers, you should have the oil changed about twice as often as the manual recommends, usually about every 3,500 miles instead of the 7,000 or so miles listed. This can extend the engine life of your car by as much as 50,000 miles.

Protect your warranty. Taking a new car to a place other than the dealership will not jeopardize your warranty. However, the station must use parts that meet the manufacturer's specifications, and you are obligated to keep accurate service records to show that you had the car serviced at or more frequently than the recommended intervals.

Take care of emissions-control systems. Federal regulations require a warranty of at least five years or 50,000 miles—whichever comes first—on emissions-control systems, even if the car changes owners. If you are having repair work done and the part is under warranty, an honest mechanic should refer you to the dealer, though you can choose not to go. The dealer is obligated to repair emissions problems for no charge if an original part or system fails due to a defect in materials or workmanship. For a complete explanation of the law, including what to do if the manufacturer will not honor your warranty claim, order a copy of "What You Should Know about Your Auto Emissions Warranty." Send 50¢ to the Consumer Information Center, Dept. 407Z, Pueblo, CO 81009.

Check the tires. Get into the habit of looking at your tires occasionally. Do any look lower than usual? How is the tread holding up? Is the tread worn more on one tire than on others? Do you see any cuts or bulges? Also, learn how to inflate your tires properly. (Don't trust the gauge on service station air pumps; they are rarely reliable. Use your own.)

hadn't marked the bulb, there was no way to tell if he had really changed it or if he had left the old one in. Either way, I paid 13 times more for a bulb I didn't need than I would have paid for the $2 fuse.

1:30 P.M. The final station I went to was in Greenwich, Connecticut. Since it was a busy shop, the mechanic warned me that it would be some time before he could look at the car. When he asked me to describe the problem, I said the car was "sort of jerky." He was a little impatient with that explanation, but I told him nothing else and left.

4:35 P.M. When I went back for the car, he explained that the problem had been a loose injector wire. His explanation was easy to follow, and he used the correct terminology. The cost: $31.16 for diagnostic time. Even though I had pretended to know nothing about cars, it didn't matter: I had found an honest mechanic.

HOW NOT TO BE A VICTIM

After my experiences, I asked Panagakos for tips on how to avoid being cheated. I had already learned that choosing a mechanic at random was not the way to go—50 percent of the service stations I went to overcharged me, whether or not I seemed knowledgeable about my car.

First of all, Panagakos maintains that your best defense is to build a long-term relationship with one good mechanic. The more you get to know him, the less likely it is that he will try to cheat you. (The trust works both ways: A mechanic who knows you may be willing to work out a payment plan if your car ever needs expensive repairs, rather than insisting on full payment immediately.)

The worst mistake most people make is bouncing from place to place: getting the oil changed at station A, going to station B to have the wheels aligned and later to station C when the car isn't running well. Instead, use the following guidelines to find an honest, knowledgeable mechanic and then stick with him. Even if your car someday has a problem that his shop doesn't handle, your mechanic should be able to refer you to a reliable place.

Ask around. Ask friends, co-workers and neighbors for references.

Check credentials. Look for a shop certified by the National Institute for Automotive Service Excellence (ASE); if you see the ASE sign displayed, go inside and ask to see the certification. You can also look for a garage certified by the Automobile Association of America (AAA); members can request a list from the local branch office.

Make sure at least one mechanic in the shop has Master Technician status (a person who is certified by the ASE in all eight categories of automotive repair). Recertification is required every five years, so make sure his is current. If you don't see the certificate displayed, ask to see it.

Ask to tour the shop. Is it well organized? Look for up-to-date equipment, including a computer analyzer.

Shop around. Ask several shops in your area for their hourly rates. Be wary of anybody who charges considerably more or less than average.

Check on the reputation. Call your local Better Business Bureau and ask if they've received any complaints about the shop you are considering.

Be prepared. Don't wait for an emergency to find out where to take your car. Do your research in advance. If you're planning a trip, have the car checked out by a mechanic you trust before you go. (If you do break down, you can still look for a shop with the certification signs explained above.)

MAINTAINING THE RELATIONSHIP

Once you've chosen a shop, there are several things you can do to ensure that you get good service every time.

Ask what the shop charges for diagnostic time. Today's cars are equipped with sophisticated computers that require equally sophisticated—and very expensive—diagnostic machinery. Make it clear that you understand you are responsible for the time it takes to do a computer analysis and find the problem.

Mechanics frequently believe that a customer will be

angry if she gets billed for a simple problem (even though it may have taken several hours to find out what was wrong). As a result, the mechanic will often change a few parts just to make the customer feel like she got something for her money. Then you end up paying for parts you didn't need in addition to the labor. (In part, I think this helps explain what happened to me in Cedar Grove, New Jersey, and Spring Valley, New York. The service stations I went to used a computer analyzer to find the loose wire.)

Describe the problem in detail. Never just say "something's wrong" and leave it at that. With a dishonest mechanic, you'll be leaving yourself open to everything from a barrage of new parts to a complete engine overhaul. (In Cedar Grove, I did describe the problem well and was still sold a bunch of unnecessary parts. But at least the parts were somewhat plausible, given the car's symptoms. What kinds of parts would he have sold me if I had acted as thought I knew nothing about cars? An expensive new water pump? A battery?)

If it means making a stupid-sounding noise, go ahead. If you feel comfortable with the mechanic, go for a test drive and indicate at what point you hear the noise. Tell the mechanic when you first noticed the problem, at what speeds it occurs, during what kind of weather (only on cold days, for example) and anything else you can think of. If you noticed fluid leaking from the car, tell him what kind: Transmission fluid is red, pink or light brown; oil can be

THE COST OF CAR REPAIRS

In this investigation, the cost of car repairs depended on the honesty of the mechanic.

Day	Headlight	Injector Wire
1	$ 2.00	$176.49
2	No charge	$ 95.33
3	$26.50	$ 31.16

amber, dark brown or black; coolant is either blue or green (a Japanese car may have red coolant). Clear water is probably normal condensation from the air conditioner.

Ask for a written estimate, especially if you don't know the mechanic well. Expect some leeway, however. Not all problems can be anticipated in advance.

Keep an eye on things. If the problem is minor and will be worked on outside the shop area, stay to watch and ask questions.

Be available. If the problem is more extensive and you cannot stay, leave a number where the mechanic can reach you. This is important because once he has found the problem, it might require your okay to fix it. If he cannot reach you, he may need to reassemble the car and move it out of the garage to make room for another car. (Ask him to give you a time frame.)

Check the evidence. Ask the mechanic to save any parts that he replaces.

Review your bill. When you get the bill, make sure everything is itemized and ask for an explanation of anything that you don't understand. Don't be intimidated by complicated-sounding terms.

—*Sharlene King Johnson*

DOWNSIZING YOUR DEBT

DEBT CAN UNDERCUT YOUR BEST-LAID PLANS FOR FUTURE PROSPERITY. HERE'S WHAT YOU NEED TO KNOW TO SHRINK YOUR FAMILY'S BILLS.

Two years ago, Kathie Anderson, a divorced 43-year-old Seattle area newspaper employee and mother of three, realized that debt was taking the joy out of her life. "I used to look forward to opening my mail," she says, "but then I started dreading it." She didn't want to face her bills.

It wasn't that Kathie was broke. She had a secure job and a decent income. The problem was the $6,800 in credit card debt she had accumulated—most of it financed at 19.8 percent interest. The interest charges alone ran to more than $100 a month, making it hard for her to ever pay off the balances. And that meant she never made much progress toward her long-term financial goals. "I knew I should be investing the money I paid for debt service instead of just throwing it away," she says.

Finally, Kathie realized that she would never get ahead unless she changed her ways and got out of debt for good. She took immediate action, liquidating $6,000 she had invested in mutual funds and retiring almost all of the credit card debt. Although her savings were wiped out, the decision, for her, was a wise one. She now has more money every month to put toward savings and investments, and there's a psychological payoff as well. "My debt reduction plan has already given me a tremendous feeling of liberation," she says.

Kathie also decided to tackle her long-term debt by paying off her 30-year $45,000 mortgage as quickly as possible. Each month, she tries to add as much as $100 to the regular $450 payment. Her goal: to own her home after 15 years. To meet that goal, Kathie will have to prepay at least $90 a month, but she will end up saving about $53,000 in interest.

Almost everyone could benefit, as Kathie has, from downsizing their debts. Nearly 16 million Americans are now experiencing some degree of difficulty in managing their debts, according to Don Badders, president of the National Foundation for Consumer Credit in Silver Spring, Maryland, and that puts them on a constant treadmill. Their financial muscle—and even their future security—is undercut by heavy interest payments. Instead of investing for the future, they're always using their cash to pay bills—or worse, to pay interest.

"Under those conditions, you may never be able to retire," says Fred Waddell, Ph.D., a family resource management specialist with the Alabama Cooperative Extension Service at Auburn University.

DO YOU OWE TOO MUCH?

Of course, making purchases on credit—which is how most people accumulate too much debt—is not inherently bad. Borrowing money and using credit can help you establish a solid credit history, and credit cards provide a convenient way to make purchases. The trouble starts when you amass debt that takes months or even years to pay off.

But how much debt is too much? One good rule of thumb: If your monthly debt payments, excluding those on the mortgage, consume 20 percent or more of your take-home pay, you're either in trouble already or close to it. "At the 20 percent level, it's often hard to pay for necessities without borrowing even more," says Tom Hufford, executive director of the Consumer Credit Counseling Service of Northeastern Indiana in Fort Wayne. "And if you don't cap it at 20 percent, it can quickly move up to 30 or 40 percent. It will get worse unless you stop borrowing." (See "Are You Headed for Financial Trouble?" on page 183.)

To find out exactly what percentage of your income is consumed by debt, take the time to total all your monthly payments. Be sure to include everything but your mortgage: the amount due every month on your loans (home equity, cars, personal or installment), overdraft checking and credit cards. Then divide the total by your monthly take-home pay. You know you're in trouble if 20 percent or more of your income is spent on debt. But even if it's not that high, you may be aghast at what you find.

"When most people look at the amounts they pay toward debt each month, they realize they could pay routine expenses with cash if they didn't have all that debt to take care of," says Karen McCall, president of Financial Recovery, a San Anselmo, California, credit and debt counseling service.

If you're not overly burdened, that's wonderful. But don't stop reading just yet. Even if your debt is manageable, you could save thousands of dollars by reducing it more quickly. For example, if you have a total debt load of around $75,000 (including a 30-year mortgage, car loans, credit cards, home-equity loan, etc.) and you can pay an extra $50 per month (that's just $1.67 a day) toward one of your obligations—keeping in mind that experts recommend you tackle the debt with the highest interest rate first—you could save about $6,000 in interest over the course of 21 years (assuming an average rate of 11 percent).

FIND HIDDEN MONEY IN YOUR BUDGET

The first step to getting debt free is simply to pay back more than the minimum amount due each month. You may feel that's impossible, especially if you're already struggling to make ends meet. But nearly any couple who tracks their spending for a month will find some surprises.

If, for example, you usually rent three movies a week and occasionally return one late, you could be spending $10 a week on video rentals without even thinking about it. That's $520 a year. Can you afford it? Is it worth it? If you're spending more than you earn, you're actually borrowing money to fund that $520 in cinematic treats, which means it's really costing you even more.

Other types of "hidden spending" that can keep you from aggressively reducing your debt include eating out (brown-bagging lunch can easily save a person from $25 to $30 a week), long-distance calls, fast-food refreshments and snacks, parking tickets and bounced-check fees. In fact, spending on such items runs so high that most credit counselors assume any family budget can be cut by 10 percent without too much pain.

EVEN THE KIDS CAN HELP

If a debt reduction plan is to succeed, everyone in the family must work together. If your husband runs up new credit card charges, that could easily negate your efforts to economize. So talk it over, and make sure he agrees that paying off debt is a top financial priority.

Next, get the children into the act. Hold a family meeting and have everyone discuss how each will contribute to the family's goal. What are their ideas for reducing spending or increasing income?

This exchange will be most productive if two steps are taken, says Flora L. Williams, Ph.D., an associate professor of consumer sciences and retailing at Purdue University in Lafayette, Indiana. First, make it clear to your children that any "austerity" program is a temporary measure. "Let them know you're going to try it for two months, then make any needed adjustments," says Dr. Williams. She also recommends linking a reward to the process—such as a day trip to a local attraction or amusement park—if everyone sticks to the plan.

To keep everyone involved, make a graph of your diminishing debts. This can be a reminder to the whole family of their achievements. If you run into trouble with the kids—perhaps your son insists on a pair of those new high-tech sneakers or your daughter must have that toy she saw on TV—avoid power struggles. "It's easier to say no if you blame 'the budget,'" says Jeanne Hogarth, Ph.D., an associate professor in the Department of Consumer Economics and Housing at Cornell University in Ithaca, New York. And "no" doesn't have to mean "nothing." It can simply mean choosing a cheaper alternative. The bottom line is that some limits must be set.

SIMPLE STEPS TO REDUCE DEBT

Once you've enlisted the help of the entire family, use some or all of the following techniques to get debt under control.

Stop incurring new debt. Rule number one is to avoid new obligations. That doesn't mean you have to cut up all your credit cards—although there are worse ideas—but it does mean that if you charge anything, you have to pay it off in full when the bill arrives. If you have an especially difficult time controlling your use of credit cards, hide them away in a safe-deposit box or a locked drawer.

Understand the true cost of credit. Before you charge anything, calculate exactly what it will cost. If you charge a $1,000 sofa on a 19.8 percent credit card and make only the minimum monthly payments, that lovely piece of furniture could end up costing you over $2,000 and take almost nine years to pay off.

Cut the rate of interest you pay. Most consumers could carry credit cards with substantially lower interest rates. In fact, you may be able to qualify for a card with a current rate as low as 9.5 percent, although you may have to pay an annual fee for the card. Other cards with slightly higher interest rates charge no annual fee. The fact is that you can almost always find a deal far better than the national average of 18.8 percent. For a listing of low-interest credit cards, check *Money* magazine or send $4 to Bank Card Holders of America, 560 Herdon Parkway, Herndon, VA 22070.

Once you receive a low-interest credit card, get a cash advance on it and pay off your other balances. *Note:* Before getting a cash advance or using one of the convenience checks that come with new cards, check to be sure the interest rate on cash advances is the same as that applied to purchases.

There are other ways to lower the rate of interest on your debt, especially with today's low mortgage rates. If you own your home, you may be able to profit from either a cash-out refinancing (you turn some of the equity in your home into cash by getting a new mortgage that's larger than your existing mortgage balance) or a home equity line of credit. For some families, such loans can be a godsend, but they must be handled with care. If you fall behind on your payments, you could stand to lose your home.

Prepay all of your debts. When used wisely, spare change can save you a fortune in interest charges, as Andrea, a 30-year-old upstate New York bookkeeper and mother of two, knows very well. Andrea and her husband, John, an excavator, save all their loose change in a plastic cereal bowl. The monthly haul is always between $20 and $30.

ARE YOU HEADED
FOR FINANCIAL TROUBLE?

Most people don't know how much they owe. They simply never stop to figure it out. But financial planners suggest that you may be carrying too much debt if:

- You are able to make only the minimum payments on your revolving charge balances.
- You use a cash advance on one credit card to make the minimum payment on another.
- You're frequently assessed late-payment fees.
- You're afraid to look at the mail.
- You're *eager* to look at the mail because it might contain an offer for a new credit card.
- You're using credit to meet ordinary living expenses.
- You're annoyed when the calendar changes each month because it signals the arrival of new bills.
- You borrow small amounts of money from friends or family for a few days.
- You borrow money in order to meet predictable expenses like insurance or taxes.
- You worry about money in the middle of the night.

If you're feeling overwhelmed by debt problems and need either professional help or an emergency solution, consider seeking advice from a nonprofit counseling service. Such agencies can set up new payment schedules with your creditors. In 1991 over 500,000 people got low-cost or free help from the Consumer Credit Counseling Service.

If you live in a rural area, it might be easier for you to get help from the Cooperative Extension Service, an educational network that combines the resources of the federal government, universities and more than 3,000 county offices. Call your local county office or a land-grant university near you for more information.

Chicken feed? Well, if you were to add just $25 to your regular payment each month on a $75,000, 30-year, 10 percent fixed-rate mortgage, you would save about $34,000 in interest—and have the mortgage paid off five years ahead of schedule. Prepaying—that is, making extra principal payments to reduce your interest charges—is effective with almost any type of loan. For most people, it's probably best to begin prepaying credit card debt. Instead of sending in the minimum amount due every month, redirect some of your spare change.

Marc Eisenson, author of *The Banker's Secret*, says there can be psychological benefits to prepaying all debts simultaneously—you feel you're running on all cylinders—rather than focusing on just one. In purely financial terms, however, the debt with the highest interest rate merits your individual attention. The choice is yours.

CONSIDER TAPPING YOUR SAVINGS

Many families shoulder heavy debt loads while also maintaining savings or investment accounts. It may be okay to regard your savings as inviolate, but you should recognize the cost of doing so: You are paying 19.8 percent interest so you can keep earning 5 percent interest in a savings account.

Some financial planners say it's not necessarily crazy to use savings to reduce debt. But the key question is: If you raid an account to pay down debt, will you be disciplined enough to pay it back? If not, you may be better off leaving your savings alone and putting aside a little each month to pay off the debt more slowly.

HOW DO YOU STAY OUT?

Downsizing debt is hard work, so most of us might assume that once we're rid of it, we'll steer clear of it. But for some people, debt springs eternal. They spend months digging out of a financial hole only to be blindsided by some unexpected expense. Then it's back into the abyss. Not surprisingly, they feel frustrated and hopeless all over again.

Such recidivism is often avoidable. You needn't stay in debt because of fairly predictable expenses. When you draw up a budget, include car repairs, medical and dental emergencies, gifts, and life and auto insurance premiums. Yes, this consistent outflow is unpleasant, but in an ideal world, you should have an emergency fund to cover the seepage.

Make a resolution right now to start a fund to cover the items that tend to drive you back into debt. If you rely on plastic for Christmas or Hanukkah, put aside $25 a month throughout the year in your own personal version of a Christmas club. Ditto for car repairs, health costs and other expenses that recur year after year. If you can't afford the full amount you should be saving for these big-ticket expenses, put aside whatever you can—and then up the ante as you retire your debts. Before you know it, you'll feel like Kathie Anderson—liberated and on the road to a secure financial future.

—Andrew Feinberg

PART SEVEN

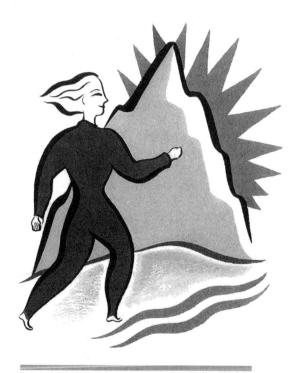

FINDING EMOTIONAL
FULFILLMENT

NO MORE BROKEN RESOLUTIONS

CHANGE IS EASY. IT'S MAINTAINING CHANGE
THAT'S HARD. HERE ARE SOME PROVEN WAYS TO
MAKE SUCCESS LAST.

In a photograph taken in the late 1950s to celebrate his first communion, my friend Bill LeBlond clutches rosary beads in tiny, ragged-looking hands. His fingernails are chewed to the quick. Bill can't remember when he started biting his nails, but he certainly remembers trying over the years to stop, never with any success. Until a day in 1981, when he was nearly 30. His girlfriend looked up from slicing onions, saw him chewing his nails and said, "That's just a habit." He never bit them again.

"It flipped a switch in my head—I could actually hear it flipping," says Bill. "I decided that if my nail biting was 'just a habit,' I could break it."

Bill told me this story a year ago on New Year's, and it stayed with me for months. If only, I thought, as I searched once again for my missing keys, change was always so simple, swift and sure—a few well-chosen words, a flash of insight and voilà, a lifetime of maladaptive behavior gone.

Psychologists who specialize in change—as well as many successful changers themselves—say it *can* happen this way. But far more often change is a marathon rather than a 100-yard dash, according to John Norcross, Ph.D., a psychology professor at the University of Scranton in Pennsylvania who has researched how people change patterns as diverse as nail biting, depression and chronic fighting with their spouses.

Dr. Norcross's research has revealed that people succeed best in sustaining change when they use a wide range of skills and supports at different points in a process that has five distinct stages. If you decide that you want to make a change in your life—whether it's as straightforward as swearing off cigarettes or as complex as leaving a dead-end career—the secret, says Dr. Norcross, is understanding exactly where in the process you are and matching that stage with appropriate strategies.

OBSTACLES TO CHANGE

First, however, it's important to understand why change is inherently so difficult. The reason, psychologists say, lies in a thicket of inertia and resistance, in personality factors as poignant as our childhood scars and as reflexive as our habits. We expect to change in a weekend, yet we have spent a lifetime becoming who we are.

Changing deeply ingrained patterns shocks our systems like a dive into icy water. Our hearts race; our lungs gasp. Our first response is to head for shore. "People are more afraid of a new pleasure than of their old familiar pain," says Olivia Mellan, a psychotherapist in Washington, D.C. "It's like an old shoe." Changing means disturbing what scientists and psychologists call homeostasis, our emotional equilibrium.

After Elly broke an old pattern of letting her boyfriend decide how they spent their time together, she reveled in her newfound assertiveness. But she also misses something her passivity gave her. "I feel a little lonely," she says. "I've lost the sense—however illusory—that someone is always looking after me."

Even when we succeed in tolerating change ourselves, we often encounter resistance from the people who love us the most. It's a nasty surprise to discover that your once-supportive boyfriend is uncomfortable when your income outstrips his or that your mother thinks you're "too skinny" when you finally manage to shed ten superfluous pounds.

"You are apt to get some powerful messages from your family not to change," says Mark Hubble, Ph.D., director of the Brief Therapy Clinic at the University of Missouri in Kansas City. "To quote a psychological proverb, 'Families operate like bureaucracies—it's a great day when nothing happens.'"

THE MOMENT OF TRUTH

In its early stages, successful change depends mostly on developing emotional awareness, says Dr. Norcross, co-author of a book on how people can change without the help of therapists. A slow, almost impalpable gathering of perception—like sand falling grain by grain onto one pan of a balance scale—precedes swift, memorable shifts into action.

According to Dr. Norcross, change often begins with a *moment of truth*, a recognition of the cost of old ways. Gloria remembers the morning when, still drunk and silly, she phoned a male friend after yet another weekend of carousing. "I love you," he told her before hanging up. "And I never want you to call me again when you're like this." Suddenly Gloria realized that her behavior wasn't sexy, wasn't charming—that she needed to get her drinking under control.

The moment of truth is only a first step. Nothing else happens without a conviction that change is possible. Something—a martial arts class, a therapy session, a talk with a friend or a quiet walk in the woods—gives successful changers a sense that life can be lived in a different way.

It was during a vacation on the Baja coast 20 years ago that Sylvia Boorstein, Ph.D., a psychotherapist in private practice in Kentfield, California, realized she could abandon a long-ingrained pattern of fearfulness. She'd stayed up worrying all through a night of crashing thunderstorms. At a trailer court near her hotel the next morning, a young woman calmly sweeping up the storm's debris smiled and told her, "My children were asleep during the storm. So I woke them up to make sure they didn't miss it."

"Before that morning, I had a thousand reasons to be a fearful person, and all the insight in the world didn't cure it," says Dr. Boorstein. "But in that moment I saw that other people live differently and that I could too."

Such a moment, when serendipity suddenly shifts the balance in our favor, is like a window opening on a spring garden. But what we *do* next—day after day, year after year—determines whether such moments produce sustained

New York State Department of Motor Vehicles
Insurance Services Bureau

ROUTING SLIP

FROM	DATE:

TO:

☐ DIAU # ☐ Pending

☐ Public Services ☐ For Hire

☐ Hearing ☐ Data Entry

☐ OFI ☐ Typing

☐ Screening ☐ Technical Support

☐ Compliance/Exceptions ☐ Other _____

COMMENTS:

_____

_____

_____

_____

_____

_____

_____

change or become meaningless memories. A leap has to be made from insight to altering your behavior in the here and now—toward your work supervisor or your mother or your lover.

Many people find that leap terrifying. They stand on the brink of action like swimmers at the edge of a cold mountain lake, temporizing, weighing the cost of change against the price of staying the same. Dr. Norcross calls this uneasy stage *contemplation.*

At this point, previously ignored inner voices may seize the microphone, strenuously arguing that change is too dangerous. These voices are as much a part of us as our drive toward progress and growth; we ignore them at our peril. This winter my friend Allison, dismayed by a photograph in which she looked sloppy and unattractive, decided to spend more time and money on her hair and clothes. But she soon realized that one part of herself was afraid of "challenging" her stylish and competitive mother, and another felt she was frivolous—shouldn't she spend that time and money helping the homeless? Her compromises: She would buy clothes for herself, but she would also start giving more money to people on the street. And she would prepare to tolerate some flak from her insecure mother.

TAKING ACTION

After contemplating the costs of action and addressing one's fears, the next step is a commitment to change. Dr. Boorstein says that after talking to the young woman in Baja, "I made an immediate vow—that I was not going to die afraid."

Psychologists say such vows work best when vague intentions—to "get in shape" or "do better at work"—are translated into concrete, realistic and achievable daily goals. "If you think you are unkind and would like to become kind, you must think exactly when, how and with whom you wish to be kind," says San Francisco psychiatrist Allen Wheelis, M.D., author of *How People Change.*

The vow is part of a stage Dr. Norcross calls *preparation,* when people test out small changes and rehearse for bigger ones. A smoker may cut down from 30 cigarettes a day to 25. A depressed woman may read an article about how to find a therapist. In this stage we search for resources, especially people who have already started to alter in themselves the same behavior we want to change, says Stephanie Brown, Ph.D., director of the Addictions Institute in Menlo Park, California. "By going to Alcoholics Anonymous, for example," she says, "a newcomer will get concrete advice, such as: 'If you drink at 5:00 every day, go for a walk at 5:00 instead.' "

For my friend Christina, the preparation stage culminated after an unpleasant night with the latest in a string of charming and unreliable men with whom she'd whiled away her twenties. In the morning, he turned to her in bed and said, "You know, I'm no good for you." She said, "You're right." When she drove away, she knew a phase of her life was over: "I had finally run out of gas on being abused."

The moment was memorable, but it followed many small efforts. "I had been slowly creating an alternative life for myself," she says. "I had stopped living alone and was happily sharing an apartment with a roommate. I was seeing a therapist. I was learning to take care of myself. Another stream was building in my life, and eventually it built up enough that I could go with it."

And so, buoyed by her stream, Christina moved into what Dr. Norcross calls the *action* stage of change. She started having lunch with a different kind of man—someone less obviously charming, someone who knew almost all her friends. Two years later, she married him.

Dr. Boorstein began to act differently as soon as she returned from Baja. One night she woke in a panic: One of her children was out late with the car. Instead of waking her husband as she usually did, she got up, made tea, took note of her catastrophic thoughts and read a magazine.

Over the course of months and years she taught herself to observe her anxieties rather than react to them, and she also began to practice meditation.

"I had to struggle," she says. "But every time I expected

disaster, I remembered that nothing terrible had happened the time before. Slowly I taught myself a new habit."

The first two weeks of taking action are the most difficult, as the old system tips into disequilibrium. Newly exercised muscles ache with tension; time once filled by smoking or overeating is suddenly, uneasily free. In Dr. Norcross's two-year study of 200 people who made New Year's resolutions, 23 percent broke them in the first week and 11 percent in the second. Then the rate slowed: Three-quarters of those who hung on for a month were still keeping their resolutions five months later.

"The first few days are torture," says Thomas Tutko, Ph.D., a specialist in sports psychology at San Jose State University in California. "After three months, the new behavior is relatively routine, and after six to eight months, it's an integral part of you."

The successful people in Dr. Norcross's study did not trust willpower alone—they made change easy on themselves in every possible way. Especially in the first rough days, they rewarded themselves—eating a favorite food after exercising, indulging in a long-distance phone call to a friend after sending out résumés to find a new job.

They rearranged their environments, throwing out cookies and half-empty cigarette packs; they put up photographs and quotes to remind themselves how they wanted to look or feel. A workaholic I know planted a terra-cotta bowl with primroses that acted as a reminder that she deserved some time out for pleasurable, purposeless contemplation.

Once a commitment has been made and action begun, the smallest details can tip the balance of competing forces in one's favor. Wearing a sleeveless, cooler T-shirt, I discovered, helps me to not slow down during my morning run. Not discussing difficult subjects when you're hungry or tired may keep you out of pointless arguments with your partner.

Dr. Norcross's study also found that successful changers reduced anxiety with activities like relaxation, meditation, exercise and healthy self-assertion. What didn't work, he found, was self-criticism: Those who lectured themselves were significantly less likely to succeed.

After the first 90 days, change enters the stage Dr. Norcross calls *maintenance.* Cravings diminish—but so does the novelty of succeeding at something new. Our friends stop remarking on our healthier bodies; they take our hard-won punctuality for granted. The weeks stretch into months, and we face another kind of test: Did we change for ourselves, or for the applause? Can we sustain our new life?

MAINTAINING CHANGE

Those who succeed at maintenance are those who don't punish themselves. A 1990 study of women who maintained weight loss found that those who allowed themselves limited but satisfying treats did far better than those who tried to live on carrot sticks—then broke down and binged on chocolate cake.

The same logic applies to other forms of behavior change. California author George Leonard, an expert on learning who also teaches the martial art of aikido, calls people who push too hard *obsessives.* "They want books, tapes and private lessons. They want to know how long it will take to get their black belts," he says. "You can write them off. They drive themselves to the point of injury and often drop out in the first month."

Leonard, who wrote *Mastery: The Keys to Success and Long-Term Fulfillment,* believes that such people have bought a cultural myth about rapid change. "Learning is not an endless series of climaxes," he says. "People need to learn to tolerate—even love—the plateaus that come between spurts of learning."

Tolerating the plateaus means accepting one's imperfections and finding pleasure in the *process* of learning. If I ran only to look good, for instance, I'd probably quit—my body won't ever be perfect. I love running for itself—for the rush in my system, the wind on my skin, the view I get of the mountain rising above my town.

At this point, finding others who are also in for the long haul—an exercise buddy, a 12-step group, a supportive lover or therapist—can mean the difference between success and failure. In Dr. Norcross's study, support networks made little difference in the first six months but were significantly helpful thereafter.

Friendly support can also help you survive a relapse—an event so common that some researchers define it as a stage of change. In Dr. Norcross's study, those who kept their New Year's resolutions reported an average of at least 14 slips during the two years. G. Alan Marlatt, Ph.D., director of the Addictive Behavior Research Center at the University of Washington in Seattle and author of *Relapse Prevention*, points out that "Alcoholics Anonymous has a saying: 'Never let yourself get too hungry, angry, lonely or tired.' That's a synopsis of relapse warning signs. The best way to fend off a relapse," he says, "is to imagine *doing* the unwanted behavior. Imagine what will happen right after you do, and what will happen after *that*, until you can picture all the results that will follow. You will usually decide that relapsing isn't worth it, and the urge will pass."

BEYOND CHANGE

Maintenance opens into a stage I call *practice*, after the term Eastern disciplines use for any lifelong activity undertaken for its own sake, rather than for immediate gain. A practice can be anything: writing, gardening, learning to sing. It need not be related to the change you've made in the previous stages. What's important is continuing to pursue your practice in all circumstances, whether or not it's raining, whether or not your lover is being supportive, whether or not you feel like it.

By following a practice we come to terms with the limits and disappointments of change. We may have learned to keep track of our keys, to develop a lean runner's body or to leave a bad relationship. But life remains difficult; its challenges do not disappear. Because a practice has no end, it is the perfect arena in which to come to terms with our imperfections.

My impulsive friend Lilly, for example, doesn't expect to become Mother Teresa by working every Sunday in her church's soup kitchen. But the weekly repetition has put her longing for change into perspective.

"I used to talk to myself so harshly," she says. "I'd say, 'You should think before you jump into things, you should be more organized, you should be more ambitious . . . .' But at the soup kitchen, a lot of my fellow volunteers are people who are over 65. Some of them are a little ditsy, some of them can't hear well. None of them are perfect, yet we couldn't run the kitchen without them. Learning to appreciate them has made me go easier on myself, too."

This kind of acceptance may be the most useful change—and the most difficult—that a person in today's change-obsessed society can ever make.

—*Katy Butler*

ARE YOU A NEGAHOLIC?

DO YOU ALWAYS EXPECT THE WORST TO HAPPEN? DO YOU BLAME YOURSELF FOR EVERYTHING THAT GOES WRONG? LEARN HOW TO STOP THAT SELF-DEFEATING BEHAVIOR AND LOOK ON THE BRIGHT SIDE.

To Joan Gregory, a 35-year-old mother of two, the job as teacher's assistant at the local elementary school sounded perfect. She interviewed with the school principal and left his office feeling pleased that it had gone so well.

But as Joan replayed the interview in her mind, her confidence waned. She had been a few minutes late because of traffic. By wanting to seem well-informed, she'd probably answered questions too quickly and seemed glib instead. And at the end of the interview, she'd dropped her purse, certainly marking her as too clumsy to handle children.

Convinced that she'd blown the interview, Joan called the

school and withdrew her application. Weeks later, she learned that the principal had been prepared to offer her the job.

Why did Joan ruin her chance at achieving an important goal? Simple: because she's a negaholic, a person who always thinks the worst—of herself, of others, of situations.

EXERCISES IN SELF-SABOTAGE

We all have days when we don't feel good or look our best, or when it seems that everything goes wrong. But while most of us are able to shrug off these unpleasant experiences, negaholics can't. "They tend to view life as a half-empty glass and focus exclusively on what's wrong with their lives," says Cherie Carter-Scott, author of *Negaholics: How to Overcome Negativity and Turn Your Life Around.* "They feel that they have no control, and they're constantly beating up on themselves."

While there are no firm figures on how many Americans suffer from negaholism, some experts believe that women are most likely to be victims. "The typical profile is a person who thinks the past was a failure, the present is miserable and the future looks bleak," says John P. Kildahl, Ph.D., a clinical psychologist and psychoanalyst in New York City and coauthor of *Beyond Negative Thinking.* "Even when something good happens, they think they'll soon pay for it with a host of unavoidable bad events."

Although negaholism may sound similar to depression, there are some key differences between the two conditions, according to Carter-Scott. While depression is a chemical imbalance, negaholism is a self-perpetuating pattern of negative thoughts that can become an addiction. Negaholics actually seem to get a perverse pleasure out of punishing themselves, says Carter-Scott. Thinking the worst allows them to avoid dashed expectations and rejection, because they think that nothing good will happen in the first place.

How does a person become such a pessimist? The condition is often the result of something that happened in childhood or adolescence. For instance, the person's parents may have had a gloomy view of life, which became "contagious." Or a failure—such as not getting into their college of choice—may have damaged the person's self-esteem to such a degree that she feels that she's worthless and that she doesn't deserve success or happiness. Finally, a trauma such as divorce or the death of a parent can also provoke a life-long pattern of self-rejection.

Eventually, negaholism begins to affect a victim's relationships. Marriages become strained, relationships with children grow tense and friends and co-workers lose patience with the negaholic's constant complaining. But no

HOW PESSIMISTIC ARE YOU?

Take the following self-test to find out whether you're a negaholic who needs to take action.

1. Do you focus on the times things didn't work out for you?
2. Do you often expect the worst so as not to be disappointed?
3. When asked what you want, do you often reply, "It doesn't matter"?
4. Do you use mistakes and mishaps in your past as reasons for not taking new risks?
5. When imagining a goal, does a voice in your head tell you that you can't accomplish it?
6. Do you find fault even with the little things you do?
7. Do you criticize yourself for what you wear, what you say, how you carry yourself?
8. Do you flog yourself with lists of things you haven't accomplished?
9. Do you have difficulty accepting compliments or celebrating achievements?
10. Looking in the mirror, are you unhappy with what you see?

Give yourself 10 points for every "yes" response. If you scored 50 or more points, you are a negaholic or well on the path to becoming one. Unless you start changing things fast, your outlook will only get worse. See "Learning to be Happy," on page 199, for techniques to help you turn your life around.

matter how frustrating the situation is, both Carter-Scott and Dr. Kildahl point out that getting angry with a negaholic only confirms her sense of worthlessness.

Instead, says Carter-Scott, "Loved ones should gently tell the negaholic how they feel when she acts this way. The person can say, 'I feel helpless when you complain. Let's think of a way to look at this differently.' It's important to separate the behavior from the person so you don't blame the victim."

LEARNING TO BE HAPPY

Fortunately, negaholics can change. Carter-Scott suggests practicing the following strategies daily.

Interrupt your negative thoughts. The more you dwell, the deeper you'll sink. Instead, busy yourself with an activity you enjoy, exercise, listen to an upbeat CD or watch a favorite video.

Stop using "must" and "should." Negaholics put pressure on themselves to do more than is humanly possible. From now on, tell yourself that you would *like* to get a new job, not that you *must.*

Stop criticizing yourself. The inner voice that's telling you that you're no good is lying. One way to silence it is to form a mental image of the voice and then realize that you can defeat it. For instance, one victim visualized the voice as a monster who wanted her to fail. She became determined to overcome it.

Write down the positive aspects of your life. Make note of all the good things you have—a job you like, lots of friends and so on—and keep a daily list of small accomplishments. You'll be amazed at how they add up and outweigh all the bad aspects.

Don't globalize problems. Avoid letting one event represent everything in your life. Not getting a promotion doesn't mean that you'll *never* get a higher-level job. Tell yourself that you'll work even harder for the next promotion. You need to look beyond one isolated disappointment.

—*Tom Clavin*

THE ROAD TO SELF-ESTEEM

THE KEY TO HAPPINESS AND SUCCESS IS GETTING RID OF ALL THOSE NEGATIVE THOUGHTS AND FEELING GOOD ABOUT YOURSELF. HERE'S HOW TO BUILD SELF-ESTEEM—AND BE A STRONGER, MORE CONFIDENT PERSON.

Money can't buy it. Success doesn't ensure it. The most unexpected women, from Princess Di to Gloria Steinem, don't have enough of it.

It's self-esteem, the catchword of the nineties. A few years ago, virtually no one talked about it; today everybody wants some. Self-esteem is being touted as the universal fix-it for women who eat, drink or love too much. It's the cure-all, experts tell us, for addictions, codependencies and other emotional problems.

WHATEVER IT IS, YOU WANT IT

But exactly what is self-esteem? The bottom-line definition: the state of feeling fine about who you are, deep down in your soul. According to the National Council for Self-Esteem (NCSE), in Sacramento, California, self-esteem is "the experience of feeling that you're worthy of happiness and capable of managing life's challenges." Less officially, it's a feel-good combination of self-confidence (having the gumption to ask for a job promotion or a raise) and self-respect (the inner grit that keeps you going, no matter what the answer).

Self-esteem is elusive, changeable, hard to get and harder to hang on to. It's an idea that's turned into an industry, spurring thousands of scientific studies in the last ten years, according to the NCSE, shelves of popular books and magazine articles and hundreds of workshops and conferences.

"Self-esteem isn't everything," says Gloria Steinem. "It's

just that there's nothing without it."

In Steinem's best-seller, *Revolution from Within: A Book of Self-Esteem*, she admits to a lifelong struggle with "inner feelings of incompleteness, emptiness, self-doubt and self-hatred."

Her confession may be the worst news yet to come out of the self-esteem movement. She's telling us that a woman of her achievements, international acclaim, outer strength and, yes, good looks, can still be drowning in self-doubt.

A NATIONAL CRISIS?

The cold, hard truth about self-esteem is that hardly anyone has all she needs all the time. The lack of it affects people in different ways. For some, low self-esteem is a roadblock to love, work, friendships and adventure. For others, like Steinem, it's a malevolent inner editor allowing them to function but deleting the joy from achievements.

It's no coincidence that Steinem's book and a gaggle of others arrived in the last year or so. We are in the midst of "a national crisis of self-esteem," says Susan Schenkel, Ph.D., a clinical psychologist in Cambridge, Massachusetts, and author of *Giving Away Success*. "As a nation and as individuals, we're apprehensive," says Dr. Schenkel. "We're not sure if we can rebuild our cities, our schools, our economy or our private lives. I see strong, confident women who are unemployed for the first time, and they are shattered. 'What's wrong with me?' they ask. They don't blame the recession; they blame themselves."

This is also the era of the recovery movement, which started in the eighties and then exploded in the nineties, with more and more support groups for alcoholics, battered women, incest survivors and victims of other traumas. "Here were rooms full of people in pain, talking about feeling bad, struggling to repair their sense of themselves," says Dr. Schenkel. "Whatever the problem, self-esteem seemed to be a large part of the cure, and that helped give birth to a new movement."

For women, self-esteem is *the* issue of the day. In the

(*continued on page* 204)

EIGHT WAYS TO BOOST
YOUR SELF-ESTEEM

1. Be realistic. "Your personal best is good enough," says Philadelphia psychiatrist Donald L. Nathanson, M.D. For instance, take the attitude of one woman who plays tennis with another woman who, she says, "is younger, stronger and faster than I am. It could be a weekly exercise in humiliation because I seldom win. Yet it's a challenge; she forces me to raise my game. If I've played well, I can walk away feeling good about myself no matter what the score."

2. Don't be materialistic. "One way to measure ourselves is by the things we have," says psychologist Maisha Hamilton Bennett, Ph.D., president of Hamilton Behavioral Healthcare, a counseling and consulting firm in Chicago. "What kind of house and car? What shape body? What color hair and eyes? To be honest, those material things can make us feel a bit better. But genuine self-esteem has interpersonal and spiritual yardsticks. Ask yourself: What do I have to give to this world? Whom do I love, and who loves me? Am I in touch with a sense of purpose in my life or a higher power?"

3. Imagine success. Even if you're not feeling confident, act as if you are, urges Dr. Bennett. Conceive it. Try to believe it. Start each morning with a vision of yourself doing all the right things at work, at play and at home. Dr. Bennett says that this works for many of her clients; champion athletes also swear by this technique of "imaging." Olympic skiers picture themselves at the top of the mountain, then speeding down it in perfect form; in other words, they mentally rehearse the act of winning.

4. Focus on your accomplishments. Each evening, review the successes you had that day, says Dr. Bennett. They can be big things—such as closing a major deal at work or running three miles for the first time—or small things, such as making a child laugh. Remind yourself of all the things you did well in communicating, relating to others, loving yourself. Look in the mirror and read your list of accomplishments aloud.

5. Take action. Set goals for yourself, advises Susan Schenkel, Ph.D., a clinical psychologist in Cambridge, Massachusetts, then figure out how to achieve them. Do you want a neater house? What room do you start with? If you want a better job, what skills do you need? How can you attain them? Get into the habit of thinking strategically.

6. Be positive. Cognitive therapy is a growing movement to help people feel better by thinking better. For instance, in divorce, self-esteem sinks. You may think, "I failed. Nothing ever works out for me. No one will ever love me again." With practice, you can learn to answer those negative thoughts with healthier ones. Write down the things that have worked out for you. Make a list of the family members and friends who do think you're worthwhile. Tell yourself that if this man loved you in the past, another man can love you in the future.

7. Meditate. Close your eyes, breathe deeply, think of peaceful, pleasant things. Then, as Gloria Steinem suggests, call up your inner child. Does she make you feel pride or shame? What's hurting her? In your deep meditation, try to imagine giving your inner child what she needs—a hug, a reassuring word, a sense of being loved. "It's never too late to have a happy childhood," says Steinem.

8. Take care of your health. Eat well and exercise often, says Dr. Schenkel. Don't let negative images lead you into neglecting yourself. One of the things that builds self-esteem is feeling strong, healthy and full of energy.

nineties, as we keep trying to have it all, many of us have reached "role overload," according to Maisha Hamilton Bennett, Ph.D., psychologist and president of Hamilton Behavioral Healthcare, a counseling and consulting firm in Chicago. "We're struggling against a backlash that blames us if we're not perfect at all our roles—marriage, child-rearing, lovemaking, working, even saving the whales. So we've got all those balls in the air—and we feel like failures if we drop just one of them."

POOR SELF-IMAGE STARTS EARLY

A growing body of research shows that many more women than men are feeling bad about themselves. According to a 1990 survey by the American Association of University Women (AAUW), from grade school to graduate school, women do as well as or better than men academically, but their self-esteem plummets over the years. When they start school, a healthy majority of both boys and girls say they are "happy the way I am." By high school, it has dropped to 46 percent for boys and only 29 percent for girls.

Girls languish in school, according to the AAUW, because they get far less attention, praise and encouragement than boys do. It may be the squeaky-wheel syndrome—noisy and restless boys demanding the teacher's attention—but being ignored and bypassed takes its toll on female self-esteem. So do puberty, sexual pressures and the effort to compete with the air-brushed, siliconed models in all those beer and blue jeans commercials.

Even the best and brightest women start to wonder about themselves. In a 1987 University of Illinois study of high school valedictorians, both sexes won good college grades, honors and scholarships. When they graduated from college, one-fourth of the men still thought they were "far above average," but none of the women would say that about themselves.

As adults, the pattern continues. Twice as many women as men suffer from severe depression. According to Donald

L. Nathanson, M.D., a prominent Philadelphia psychiatrist and author of *Shame and Pride*, classical depression (one kind of severe depression) is linked to weepiness, morbid thoughts about the future and guilt (bad feelings about what you've done).

Atypical depression, another type of severe depression, which is more common than its name suggests, is linked to low self-esteem or deep shame (bad feelings about who you are.) Outwardly, some people with this form of depression seem to be functioning well, but they are haunted by an inner bleakness. This is the form of depression that didn't respond to traditional medications, but doctors are now reporting good results with the drugs Prozac and the newer Zoloft.

FALSE PERCEPTIONS ABOUND

For many women, the trait that blossoms from low self-esteem is self-criticism—especially of their bodies. In one psychological test, people are shown an array of body silhouettes, ranging from skeletal to obese, and asked to pick the one that's closest to their own.

No matter what they actually weigh, men tend to pick a silhouette that's two or three sizes thinner. Women, whether they're anorexic, normal or overweight, point to a silhouette two or three times larger.

"The typical man always thinks he's this side of Robert Redford," explains Carol Burger, Ph.D., director of the Women's Research Institute at Virginia Polytechnic Institute and State University in Blacksburg. "And the typical woman, trying to live up to all those media images, never thinks she's thin enough or good enough."

That out-of-focus body image was part of Steinem's problem. Men pursued her, and other women wanted to look like her, copying her clothes, her aviator glasses, her cascade of long hair. All along, she was squinting in the mirror and seeing the forlorn "pudding-faced" child she used to be.

Like so many things, self-esteem goes back to childhood. Most of us start off with a good supply of it. But even as babies, while every little success builds up our self-esteem, every little failure can chip away at it. "For a little child, success or failure is in the eye of the beholder—the parent," explains Dr. Nathanson. "The trouble is that on a scale of 1 to 10, some parents want to behold a 12.

"Some measure their child by an imaginary ideal. Others just can't help comparing her or him to other children. Who walks or talks sooner? Who's prettier? When she lives up to the parent's ideal, the child feels pride, the emotion of healthy self-esteem. When she falls short, she feels shame, a sense of being defective and unlovable, the emotion of low self-esteem."

As we move through life, the comparisons continue. So does the need for approval—and the struggle to hang on to our self-esteem. "Think of self-esteem as a moving point on an axis," suggests Dr. Nathanson. "It's the distance between your ideal self and the self you see at this moment."

The trick, he says, is to see both these selves clearly. Some people, like Steinem, underestimate their current selves, and so the gap seems wide and full of shame. Others overestimate the ideal. Is it your personal best, tailor-made to your own desires and abilities, a goal you can realistically chase after? Or is it a false idol, hammered together with all the "oughts" and "shoulds" from parents and teachers, friends and employers, lovers and fashion ads?

HOW TO FEEL BETTER ABOUT YOURSELF

The first step on the long, winding road to self-esteem is to take a personal inventory. Dr. Nathanson urges his patients to make as long a list as possible of their positives, both big and small. Can you operate a VCR? Are you raising two wonderful children? Are you a good neighbor? A hard worker? A faithful friend?

When something goes wrong—whether it's a social gaffe, a missed job promotion, a lost love—consult that list. "That way," says Dr. Nathanson, "you can isolate the event. You can see it as a specific experience, not something that defines your whole life. You can look at it as a particular failing, one trait among many others, an individual mistake that is part but not all of you.

"The cure for low self-esteem is to be specific about what has happened," he continues. "Are you crestfallen? Head bowed? Longing to run and hide? You can deny it, get angry, try to drown it in drink or food. Or you can name the feelings and face the flaw that's been exposed. Then, instead of giving up on yourself, you can think about what you need to change and how you want to improve."

Once you've admitted those painful feelings, chase them away by doing something nice for yourself, Dr. Nathanson says. Treat yourself to lunch with a friend who cares for you—and lets you know it. Start a new hobby or take a course—something that will give you a small taste of success, giving you a dose of "situational self-esteem," as therapists call it.

Bouts with self-doubt are part of life, and with time, most of us get over them. For some people, though, low self-esteem is chronic, as nagging as a toothache, as persistent as cellulite. "Some people may have a chemical imbalance, and they are the ones who need medication to help them through their remorseless, shame-loaded depression," says Dr. Nathanson. "Many others, though, can be helped by talking with a caring spouse or friend or therapist. Perhaps they grew up in a shaming, name-calling family. Perhaps they had a series of bad experiences or a single great trauma that hasn't been worked through.

"These people need to confront their experiences and process them. Perhaps they'll find the mistake they made, confusing a single experience with a global view of themselves. Perhaps they'll learn to see themselves more clearly, both who they are today and who they want to grow up to be."

All of the steps toward better self-esteem begin by taking some action. That can mean changing your thought patterns, your surroundings, even the people around you.

To make positive changes in her life, Steinem had to end

a love affair that required her to be less than herself. To feel more deserving, she redecorated her apartment, changing it from a crash pad to a real home. In midlife, she underwent treatment that let her get rid of the glasses she'd been hiding behind since sixth grade. At the same age, another woman, depressed about the progress of her career, went back to school to pursue an MBA.

"That's self-esteem," says Dr. Nathanson. "It's the courage to act, even if you may fail, even if you may humiliate yourself all over again. The real shame is to do nothing."

—*Claire Safran*

HOW TO MAKE DECISIONS YOU WON'T REGRET

EVER ENVY THOSE WOMEN WHO SEEM TO MAKE THE RIGHT CHOICE EVERY TIME? YOU CAN DO IT, TOO. IT'S A MATTER OF TUNING IN TO YOUR PERSONAL RADAR.

A woman who's just lost her job feels a strong impulse to walk into a local health club. A membership is the last thing she can afford, but the urge is peculiarly insistent. While giving her a tour, the sales manager tells her the club is looking for a receptionist. She applies for the job and gets it.

Another woman meets her husband's new boss, a successful attorney, for the first time. He's well-dressed and cordial—but when she shakes his hand, her skin crawls. Her husband is so enthusiastic she shrugs off her misgivings. The attorney turns out to be unethical. Her husband hates working for him.

We've all had experiences like these: times when we loved or hated someone at first sight without knowing why; when we felt inexplicably compelled to go someplace—or *not* to go; when we sensed what was going to happen before it did.

DON'T MINIMIZE INTUITION

The times we've heeded these instinctive gut reactions and they've turned out to be right—enabling us to avoid danger, seize an opportunity, help someone we care about—are among the most powerful experiences of our lives. At these moments we feel mysteriously guided, whether by a higher power or by our own personal radar.

And it's not just you and I who have noted intuition's powers. "Today intuition is being taken much more seriously by the very people you would think would pooh-pooh it—the business community," says Philip Goldberg, author of *The Intuitive Edge: Understanding Intuition and Applying It in Everyday Life*. "They are recognizing it as an important component of decision-making and problem-solving."

Unfortunately, we don't always read our radar correctly. Sometimes a gut message is one that we're just not ready to hear yet. We shrug it off as "just my imagination." When it later turns out to be true, we want to kick ourselves.

More confusing are the times when we get a strong gut feeling and follow it—straight into trouble. We fall deeply in love with someone who turns out to be painfully wrong for us; we bet our nest egg on a hunch and lose it. When this happens, says Goldberg, it's not that our intuition is wrong, it's that we've mistaken something else for intuition. "The dictionary defines *intuition* as 'knowing directly, without the use of rational processes,' " Goldberg observes. "*Knowing*—not guessing. Intuition is something that turns out to be true."

Misleading messages from our gut, by contrast, concern something we *want* to be true ("I just know he's the right man for me," because you're lonely or the biological clock is ticking) or *afraid* is true ("I just know something has happened because he's never late.") A wish or a fear appears on the radar screen and we mistake it for a fact.

"They're easy to confuse," says Philadelphia psychotherapist Judith Sills, Ph.D., because wishes and fears, as well as
true intuitions, "can come with strong, compelling feelings—
and without logic."

How then can we learn to distinguish better between
gut reactions we should pay attention to and ones we should
ignore? And must we always wait for intuition to visit us, or
can we call on it when we need its help?

An accurate sixth sense can make a dramatic difference
in our relationships, our career, our finances—it can even
save our lives. Businessman Ray Kroc bought the budding
McDonald's fast-food chain against the expert advice of his
consultants because "I felt in my funny bone it was a sure
thing." Actress Sophia Loren once canceled her appearance
at a charity ball because of "an overwhelming feeling of
impending disaster." The plane she would have been on
crashed, killing everyone on board.

THE BRAIN/GUT REACTION

Scientists don't yet know what happens in the brain
when we have a gut intuition. Even quantum physics can't
explain how we receive information across time and space:
how Sophia Loren could have sensed a plane crash that
hadn't happened yet—an example of what she calls her
"acute extrasensory perception."

But not *all* gut intuitions are necessarily psychic, says
Goldberg. What feels like a flash of ESP may sometimes be a
"very rapid interference" from data our senses have picked up
"subliminally"—below the threshold of awareness.

At a happy family reunion, Gina Monroe-Beaupré of
Duluth, Minnesota, saw her 77-year-old father across the
room and "suddenly his face faded away from me. I had a
compelling urge to go to him. I knelt down and put my head
in his lap and said, 'I love you. I'm scared of when you die.' "
It was the last time she saw him; he died six weeks later of a
massive heart attack. Psychic? Or did she sense a subtle
change in her father's energy level or color?

Driving on the Los Angeles Freeway, Margaret Pearson

jammed on her brakes and put on her flashers a moment *before* the motorcyclist in front of her went down. "I think I saved his life!" she says. Psychic? Or did Pearson pick up tiny clues that the rider was in trouble?

When we take an instant, "irrational" dislike to someone, are we being psychic—or are we accurately reading body language? One thing is for sure: In the words of neurophysiologist Paul MacLean, M.D., chief of brain evolution and behavior at the National Institute of Mental Health in Rockville, Maryland, "The brain is smarter than we are."

There's a widespread popular belief that intuition lives in the right side of the brain, but several top brain researchers say this theory is simplistic and inaccurate. It's "an attempt to find an easy answer to . . . a fantastically complicated function," explains Richard Davidson, Ph.D., professor of psychology and psychiatry at the University of Wisconsin in Madison.

A gut intuition probably involves many parts of the brain working together. It's the limbic system, where moods and emotions originate, that accounts for the *gut* in *gut reaction*. "The limbic brain is the main mind/body transducer," explains Laurie Nadel, psychologist and coauthor of *Sixth Sense*. "Nearly all of your physiological processes are regulated there." When your cerebral cortex picks up important information, "it may signal the limbic system, and you may experience a physical sensation or an emotion that you describe as 'a gut feeling' or 'a sixth sense.'"

Psychologist/philosopher Eugene Gendlin, author of *Focusing*, confirms that the most common place in which we sense the truth is our stomach. Other sensations that were reported to Philip Goldberg include "tightening up," "quickening heartbeat," "a glow," "a burning sensation," "a chill," "prickling," "tingling," "electricity running through me."

These responses are highly individual. "Your own intuition is unique," says Nadel. No one can describe how your feelings will signal you, but if you can recall how you feel when you have a gut reaction, you'll begin to recognize your own signaling system. "Keep a list of your intuitive experiences and note any identifying characteristics," Nadel suggests. Does the message come in words, visual images or just a feeling? What happens in your body? You may not necessarily be able to describe your signals verbally.

IS IT A TRUE GUT REACTION?

Confusion occurs because the limbic system, so closely linked to intuition, is also activated by wishes and fears—things that really *are* all in your mind. Since these too can be accompanied by a churning stomach, pounding heart or chills, how can we tell the difference? Intuitive signals may be more specific and localized. "Intuition tends to make itself felt in a particular part of the body rather than spreading across a wide area, as anxiety or panic does," says Nadel.

Sometimes the sheer power or nagging insistence of a gut reaction is enough to distinguish it from everyday emotions. As a young man in communist Romania, my husband's best friend, Ernie Kugler, was living and working illegally in a different town from his family. Getting caught would have meant a sentence of forced labor. He had reason to be scared all the time. Yet just once he had "a colossal feeling" that, as he puts it, "I absolutely *had* to go home. I had no idea why, but I went." That night at 2 A.M., the police knocked on his family's door for a spot check. Kugler was in his bed.

When it's not clear whether your gut's in the grip of fact or fantasy, "let novelty be your guide," advises Dr. Sills. Real information, however it comes to us, is new and unexpected; fantasy is all too familiar. It falls into patterns we can recognize. "If you *know* you're phobic about flying, then your anxiety attack on the way to the airport is not intuition," says Dr. Sills. The time to pay attention, she advises, "is when you say, 'I don't know where this feeling is coming from. This is not typical of me.'"

Another technique is to ask, "Which came first, the message or the feeling?" It's a subtle difference, but in a true gut reaction, the emotion is a *response* to information, while an emotion is the driving force that *creates* impostor reactions.

"Maybe you can't say to yourself, 'I'm scared to go to this

party,' " says Sills. "So what you say is, 'I have a bad feeling; I'd better not go.' When your inner voice tells you no, review it: Is that really a 'No, I'm scared'? Or is it 'No, for reasons that I can't pinpoint—it's just a sense I have'? If it's the second example, listen."

"As much as I advocate intuition," Goldberg says, "I also advocate putting it to the test: Gather facts, think rationally, get other opinions. Whenever possible, check things out—especially when your emotions are involved, when there's a lot at stake or when it's in an area where you've made mistakes before."

In choosing a day-care center, for instance, you may ricochet between the need for child care and the fear of child abuse. Listen to your gut—but check credentials and talk to other parents, too.

Everyone's intuition is stronger in some areas than in others. Where your track record is poor, don't trust your gut at all. For example, if you've swooned over a string of rotten men, you'll want to put your latest infatuation to the test before you start making wedding plans.

FOUR WAYS TO FOSTER INTUITION

"You can no more force intuition than you can force someone to fall in love with you," Goldberg writes. But, "you can prepare yourself for it, invite it and create attractive conditions to coax it." You can even ask for its help with a specific problem. Here are some ways to help you make your gut a trustworthy guide.

Believe. "It helps to believe that your mind can work on levels you're not in touch with and that unusual insights and remarkable illuminations can come from *you*," Goldberg says.

Break set. Rigid, habitual patterns of thought and behavior can shut out intuition. "Question your assumptions and beliefs," Goldberg suggests. "Take a different route to work. Read a wider range of books and magazines. Talk to people you think you have nothing in common with. Expect the unexpected."

Practice. Exercise your intuitive muscles. Some of Goldberg's methods: "Practice making quick, ten-second decisions on minor matters, like ordering from a menu or deciding what to wear. Make predictions, going with the first thought that comes to mind: Who's calling when the phone rings, who will win the ballgame. After brief meetings with strangers, try to imagine their lives and personalities," then check out your hunches.

Dr. Sills believes that the best way to strengthen your intuitive voice is through visualization—controlled daydreaming where, with eyes closed, you imagine you're eating a peach or walking on the beach. "Mental imagery techniques are about opening the channel to the problem-solving, understanding part of your brain," says Dr. Sills.

Relax. "Anxiety and stress work against intuition," Goldberg says. Yet we all tense up in the midst of knotty problems and tough decisions—when we need intuition's help the most. "When you feel stuck," says Goldberg, "get away for a while. Put your mind on something else. Take a walk, a nap, a vacation." The answer may just flash in your mind.

According to Jose Silva, creator of the Silva Method—a system for tapping the brain's natural powers—learning to relax at will is the key to intuition. When we relax, our brain waves enter the slower, more regular alpha frequency, known to be associated with creativity, ESP and meditation. Here are some relaxation techniques from the Silva Method.

- Sitting comfortably in a chair or lying down on the bed, close your eyes. Then take a deep breath. As you slowly exhale, say to yourself, "Relaaaax."
- Using all your senses, imagine a tranquil beach or forest.
- Let your awareness travel slowly through your body from head to toe, relaxing each part, inside and out: scalp, forehead, cheeks, throat, shoulders, chest, etc.
- Relax your eyelids. Let that relaxed feeling flow down through your entire body.

- Count down slowly from 50 to 1. Then say to yourself, "Every time I relax this way I go deeper, faster."

Using one or more of these techniques from one to three times a day for 5 to 15 minutes will reduce stress and invite more intuition into your life.

"Intuition is a mental activity that *can* be nurtured and cultivated," declares Nadel. Activated by your trust, fine-tuned by your attention, this amazing guidance system in your brain will lead you more surefootedly through life.

—Annie Gottlieb

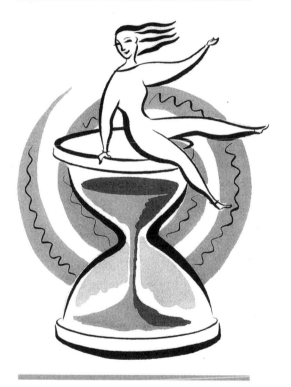

PART EIGHT

TIME JUST FOR YOU

TIME FOR YOU: ALONE

TO CENTER YOURSELF, TIME ALONE IS ESSENTIAL.
WHETHER IT'S FOR A HALF HOUR OR A FULL DAY,
WOMEN NEED TO FIND A LITTLE TIME WITHOUT
INTERRUPTION—OR GUILT.

While she was growing up, Barbara, a nutritionist, shared a room with her sister—and yearned for a little privacy, a space of her own. Now Barbara is a mother of two with a loving physician for a husband. She's still yearning for a little private space.

When she and Gordon were first married, she got a few nights a week to herself when he was on call at the hospital. That worked well. But when the children were born, her private moments ended.

"I'm never alone now at home," she complains. "And I really need to be—to read, take walks, to just think. When I don't get any time by myself, it makes me tense."

She remembers one incident in particular. Gordon had taken their two sons out grocery shopping one night. "I figured I was all set for 45 minutes, maybe even an hour," she says. But about 10 minutes later—after she had joyously settled down with a cup of decaf and a long-awaited novel—she heard the garage door open. Gordon had forgotten his checkbook, and rather than simply picking it up and going back out, he called off the entire shopping trip. Says Barbara, "I went from total contentment to absolute resentment; my private time was over before it began."

Barbara is not alone in suffering from privacy deprivation. It's a dilemma that many women face these days with the demands of career, child-rearing, family, friends and community responsibilities.

What exactly is privacy deprivation? It's the opposite of being lonely. It's when you sneak off with a sandwich and a magazine, and you hear, "Mom, I'm hungry." It's when you come home exhausted after a tyrannizing day at work and your partner demands some attention, or a friend or relative calls with a problem. It's being overstimulated by people, noise and everyday problems—and not finding a moment or place to concentrate, refresh yourself or experience some enjoyment all by yourself.

WHERE HAS YOUR PRIVACY GONE?

Raymond Flannery, Jr., Ph.D., stress researcher at Harvard Medical School and author of *Becoming Stress Resistant*, observes that after working and sleeping we have about 62 hours left in the week for leisure, cultural and community pursuits and personal time—which includes everything from eating, exercising, getting dressed, paying bills and seeing the doctor to taking care of the children (if you work full time), getting the car fixed and taking the car back to the garage when it still doesn't run right. Obviously, not much time gets to be spent alone. "Privacy time, though, has to be worked into your schedule," says Dr. Flannery. "You can't ignore your need for privacy and stay healthy."

The problem is that we've begun to think of privacy as an expendable luxury, not as a *need*. Harriet B. Braiker, Ph.D., author of *The Type E Woman (How to Overcome the Stress of Being Everything to Everyone)*, says, "[Certain] high-achieving women are imploded with demands, both external and internal, and lack the skills to filter them. These women complain that the first thing they sacrifice is their private time or private pleasures." In fact, this phenomenon affects almost all working women, *especially* lower-paid working mothers.

Although domestic equality has improved somewhat over the past 20 years, women (including those who work outside the home) are still responsible for twice as much household maintenance and three times as much child care as men, says Geoffrey Godbey, Ph.D., professor of leisure studies at Pennsylvania State University in University Park. When women do seek time out, they're usually still "on call," he says. "Women's time is much more easily interrupted than men's time."

Dr. Godbey points out that a man will say, "I'm going to

sit down and read," and he does it. But a woman will say, "I'd like to read if . . . the kids are okay, the dishes are put away and the bills are paid."

You don't have to be married or a mother, of course, to experience privacy deprivation. Diane, who lives alone, gets exhausted between dating her boyfriend, Michael, her private social work practice and trying to stay in touch with her women friends. "I'll be on the sofa under a blanket, reading, with a cup of coffee nearby. It'll be great—and then Michael will call. He'll suggest we go bike riding because it's such a nice day. And I may go, even though I don't want to: It interferes with my schedule of being alone," she admits.

Many women like Diane tend to put others' needs before their own. Our culture has said women are meant to nurture. Rather than disappoint someone else, we give up our privacy.

LACK OF SOLITUDE TAKES ITS TOLL

When we don't get the time to recharge our batteries, the result is privacy deprivation, a prime source of negative stress. According to Dr. Braiker, chronic overarousal taxes your body and leads to fatigue and depletion of the immune system.

In *Becoming Stress-Resistant*, Dr. Flannery explains how stress can lead to physical illness. His book is based on his findings in a 12-year study of 1,200 men and women attending a night-school program who underwent a lot of stress studying, working during the day and raising families.

Dr. Flannery measured their stress level by the frequency of their illnesses. The students who didn't take time out for relaxation reported more illnesses than those students who did. One of the most important reasons, says Dr. Flannery, is that those students who couldn't find private time to relax during some part of every day neglected other personal needs, such as exercise and good nutrition, too.

Privacy-deprivation stress will also harm your emotional well-being, causing resentment, burnout, moodiness and depression. And, naturally, your relationships with your family and friends will suffer. Says Barbara, "When I haven't been alone for a while, the kids start to annoy me. And I don't feel like being intimate with Gordon; sex doesn't appeal to me unless I'm rested and have had some time to myself."

GIVING SOME TIME TO YOURSELF

Your need for privacy depends on your personality and lifestyle. Introverts usually require more privacy than extroverts. People who work alone may desire privacy less than those who are surrounded by others the whole day. Privacy needs can also change according to your life circumstances. If you're in mourning, you may need more time by yourself. Whatever your situation, here's how to work some privacy into your life.

Give yourself permission to seek privacy. Recognize that it's a *priority* you owe to your health and well-being to meet. Anthony Storr, M.D., psychiatrist at Oxford University in England, writes in his book *Solitude*, "Removing oneself voluntarily from one's habitual environment promotes self-understanding and contact with those inner depths of being which elude one in the hurly-burly of day-to-day life."

Decide what privacy means to you. The time to read a whole chapter in a book? Watching the news with no interruptions? Or maybe it's just staring at the ceiling while you drift off. Whatever it is, commit yourself to getting the type of privacy you need.

Scrutinize your daily schedule and ask yourself "Where can I cut back?" Look at your calendar a week or two in advance and keep a few lunches free for yourself. Also, plan something special for yourself when your child has a slumber party to attend or your partner has a business trip.

Establish—and stick to—a privacy routine. Pick a time and place when and where you won't be interrupted except for emergencies. Maybe it'll be in the tub for a half hour after work. Or for a walk right after breakfast on

Saturday. Declare this to *everyone* who usually makes demands on your privacy time.

Barter with your spouse, neighbor or friend for privacy time. Dr. Godbey suggests using each other to take care of the kids, and make sure that your privacy partner assumes all responsibilities (except for crises) that arise during your absence.

Be creative. Make all necessary arrangements with your family, and then check yourself into a nice local hotel room for a night.

If you're a mother, occasionally eat a meal away from the kids, and taste your food for a change. Go to bed an hour earlier than your companion and stretch out all by yourself. Take a drive or work in your garden.

Teach others—your friends, your children—about the rewards of privacy. Do this by respecting *their* needs for privacy, and they'll learn that giving oneself quality time benefits everyone.

—Ilene Springer

EXERCISE FOR FUN (FOR A CHANGE)

TIRED OF THE SAME OLD AEROBICS CLASS?
LOOKING FOR A NEW WAY TO WORK OUT?
HERE'S A LOOK AT THE HOTTEST
NEW FITNESS TRENDS.

Call it Repetitive Sweat Syndrome. Even for those dedicated women who relish exercise, flogging their bodies in the same fast-paced aerobics class five times a week can lead to boredom and burnout. When the instructor begins to resemble a ball and chain swathed in Lycra, fitness experts say it's time to look for alternatives.

In fact, doctors and trainers stress that variety in exercise is not just the spice of a healthy life, it's the main course. Indeed, exercise has diversified. Alternatives to aerobics range from traditional boxing workouts in formerly all-male gyms to yoga classes in darkened rooms perfumed with incense and fresh flowers. Aerobics itself has blossomed into dozens of dance, swimming and weight-training—inspired varieties. And for women who get antsy at the very thought of sweating within four walls, clubs are offering Roller-blading (excuse us, in-line skating) and power-walking classes that turn the great outdoors into a cross-training circuit. And that's just the start.

SWEATING THROUGH GYM CLASS

Women are turning to traditional neighborhood gyms, where workout clothes are more like Stanley Kowalski T-shirts and pull-up bars stand in lieu of Stair-Masters. There they skip rope, spar with punching bags, do sit-ups and lift weights.

"Women are going to gym classes, doing push-ups and squat thrusts—all the things high-powered athletes have never gotten away from," says veteran trainer Tina de Lemps. And there's usually a good gym in every city. In Chicago, a colorful, no-nonsense gym is Fima's Russian Fitness. "This is a serious gym for serious people," says owner Fima Feigin. "This is a Russian gym. You come, you lift weights and work out, lose some body fat, gain a little muscle and go home. There's no singing and dancing."

BOXING FOR A BEAUTIFUL BODY

For a rigorous, no-frills workout, many women are boxing, blowing off a little steam along with the calories. "It's one of the best exercises you can do," says Jay Bialsky, a physical therapist and owner of Medi-Worx, a sportsmedicine clinic in New Jersey. "Boxing increases strength and burns fat at the same time." At Gleason's Gym in Brooklyn, women (who make up nearly 30 percent of new members) are training alongside aspiring contenders, matching their sweat drop for drop. In the vast, old-fashioned gym that smells of perspiration, old leather and dust, members do 90-minute workouts one-on-one with a trainer, jumping rope, jabbing at punching bags, sparring in rings and puffing through one-handed push-ups.

"They train three minutes, then rest one minute, then train three minutes, and so on—just like rounds of boxing," says Bruce Silverglade, Gleason's owner. "It's a complete cardiovascular workout, and you're working your upper and lower body. You're also learning the sport of boxing, so you're getting speed and agility. Boxers have to be fast." What appeals most to women members, says Silverglade, apart from strength and confidence, is the lean, graceful body a boxing workout promotes. "You get long, thin muscles, like a dancer's or a long-distance runner's, as opposed to bulky muscles, like a weight lifter's."

BEYOND BOXING

Michael Olajidé, Jr., a former middleweight contender, has taken the boxing workout out of the ring and into the aerobics classroom with Aerobox at the Equinox gym in New York City. Olajidé leads his students through a grueling hour of nonstop rope-skipping, sliding and jabbing that quickly leaves them drenched and red-faced—all to the beat of Chaka Khan and techno-house.

"It's aerobics gone hard-core," says Olajidé. Proponents of Aerobox and similar boxing-cum-aerobics classes around the country (like Executive Boxing at Bodies in Motion in Los Angeles) praise the upper-body workout that many aerobics classes don't provide. Lunging and ducking imaginary punches work the lower body and legs. "The flavor of Olajidé's class is boxing, drilling. It's like boot camp," says Lavinia Errico, co-owner and program director of Equinox. "In Aerobox, there's no time to stop." Indeed, at Olajidé's breakneck pace, there's barely time to breathe.

Karate, too, is becoming more of a workout. In his Seido karate classes at Apex in Manhattan, Erroll Bennett eases newcomers into the idea with a buddy system, letting seasoned students shadow novices. Intensive squatting and repetitive kicking exercises give the hips, thighs and calves a burning workout, and yes, the chopping motions give arm muscles strength and definition.

Just as boxing begat Aerobox, so Aerobox begat Double Dutch Duke, a jump-rope class also offered at Equinox. Instructor Kacy Duke drew her inspiration from the long, sweaty jump-rope sessions in Olajidé's class. If Aerobox is boot camp, Double Dutch Duke is a playground for grownups. After a series of rope-jumping exercises, abdominal work and calisthenics, the class closes with a big communal jumping session with room-length ropes. "Jumping rope works your arms, your tush, your quads, your wrists and your coordination. You feel it all over," says Equinox's Errico.

FUNK AND HIP-HOP

For exercisers who favor a ropeless workout and secretly harbor dreams of becoming a Sir Mix-a-Lot dancer, aerobics has spawned dozens of funk and hip-hop dance classes that blend street-inspired dance moves into an aerobics format.

In his Funky Fitness classes at Jeff Martin and Molly Fox studios in New York, instructor Michael Stephens leads aspiring fly girls through a slow, hip-thrusting warm-up. Then, to the thump of house-music standards like Snap's "I Got the Power" and Bobby Brown's "Humpin' Around," he breaks down choreographed steps, practices them with the class and then speeds it up. At the end of the hour, even newcomers are jumping, spinning and strutting their way through the dance, executing fairly convincing pivot-dip combos à la Hammer.

The biggest draw of these classes, says Stephens's teaching partner, Annie Niland, "is the fun factor. If someone enjoys dancing, they'll stick with the workout, and that's where the fat burning comes in. People tell me funk changed their bodies." Sports therapist Bialsky warns of the potential dangers of combining step and funk classes. "If you're executing a complicated twist on a step, you're not on stable ground. You can overshoot the step. We see a lot of twisted ankles from those classes."

The popularity of dance-flavored aerobics has given rise to a virtual dinner-length menu of classes—with lots of ethnic choices thrown in. At Valerie Green's Afro-Dynamics class at Prescriptive Fitness in New York, live drummers lead a class that combines low-impact aerobics with West African, Haitian and Brazilian dance techniques. Vigorous upper-body movements work the torso and arms. At Main Street dance studio in Santa Monica, students in the Swing Brazil class learn samba steps spliced with low-impact aerobics to the beat of live percussion. Niland draws her choreographic inspiration from the African and Brazilian dances she sees on the Discovery channel. She says, "African-based dance, like funk and samba, keeps the body low to the ground, so the quads and butt get a strenuous workout."

NO-IMPACT AQUA-AEROBICS

Another burgeoning aerobics spin-off provides a perspiration-free workout in an injury-free environment. Aqua-aerobics, available now at most gyms equipped with pools, has long been a favorite of physicians and physical therapists because there's no impact involved. In Sherri Ehrlich's Power Plunge classes at the Vertical and T.S.I. clubs in New York, students do a 30-minute aerobic workout by kicking, jogging and lunge-walking up and down the length of the pool, followed by a 15-minute strength-training session.

Ehrlich uses Hydro-tone equipment—bright yellow boots and dumbbells bristling with plastic wings that increase resistance: The faster students move their arms and legs in circles and arcs, the more weight they move. At the Fontainebleau Spa in Miami Beach, dozens of aqua-aerobics classes are given every week. The instructors use blue plastic AquaBells, which cup the water and create weight, as well as plastic jugs filled with water for exercises that strengthen the back and arms.

For women who want to burn fat and lose weight, says Elliott Hershman of the Nicholas Institute of Sports

Medicine, pool exercise requires some extra effort. "Because the water cools your body as you exercise, you have to work really hard to get your core body temperature to the point where you burn calories," he explains.

CYCLING SPIN-OFFS

For those who bought a stationary bike dreaming of a Tour de France competitor's body and found only ennui and a flaccid upper torso, many gyms are now offering classes that inject new life into an old idea. In Cathy Yelverton's Bikercize class at the Eastern Athletic Club in Brooklyn, students work the upper body with weights and Dynabands while pedaling stationary bikes.

Biking classes that engage the upper body, however, aren't a favorite of physiotherapists. "When you're on a bike moving your upper and lower body, you're basically unstable," says Bialsky. "Something's going to take the stress, and it's most likely going to be the back."

Johnny G.'s Spinning class at Voight Fitness and Dance studio in Los Angeles simulates a long outdoor bicycle workout—not much arm work, but a grueling session for the legs. Johnny describes hills, potholes and other obstacles to each member over individual headsets, and the rider responds both intellectually, by imagining the course, and physically, by adjusting the tension on the bike.

"Spinning is a hard-core, very mental workout," says fitness instructor Karen Voight. "The idea is to relax under stress and increase your performance level as the tension builds." But students say that if Johnny's not leading the class, an hour on a bicycle seat dodging imaginary potholes is as much fun as changing a real flat tire.

MOVING TO THE GREAT OUTDOORS

Exercisers who like to use their wheels outside can join Rollerblading classes like those at Crunch Fitness in Manhattan. These classes get the uninitiated up and rolling, and for the advanced blader they demonstrate how to get the most aerobic and anaerobic exercise out of a session. The trick, says Carl Foster, a director of sports science for the U.S. Speedskating Association, is to use your heart as a guide. At about 160 beats a minute, an average woman skater could get a workout comparable to a good run.

For those who are wary of workouts that require wheels, new classes offer an old trick: walking. Apex offers a power-walking class in Central Park, where students do push-ups and tricep work on park benches and lunge-walk up hills as part of a vigorous, speedy 60-minute walk.

The Reebok Bodywalk Program was pioneered at the Boston Athletic Club. Walkers do a five-mile loop on Castle Island, using park benches for isometric work and hills for sprint-walking and lunge-walking. Reebok will soon offer the walking curriculum on video and on audio tape. "Brisk walking is probably the simplest, safest workout you can find outside a gym," says Kathie Davis, executive director of IDEA, a fitness professional organization. But *brisk* is certainly the operative word: "You have to go fast enough to raise your heart rate to about 60 to 85 percent of your target rate," says Apex's Carol Espel, an exercise physiologist who designed the club's walking class. Espel notes that walking is a good calorie burner as long as it's kept up for at least 20 minutes, and ideally 40 to 60 minutes for real fat burning. "As for overall tone," she adds, "it's great for the lower body. And it's virtually injury free as long as you've got a good pair of shoes."

THE NEW, OLD YOGA

The new alternatives to aerobics aren't necessarily all new. At health clubs, exercisers with high-stress jobs are opting out of high-impact, high-noise classes for a quiet hour of yoga. "It's the one place many people find where they can concentrate on their bodies, but they don't have to be competitive," says Lora Holbrook, a yoga instructor for T.S.I. clubs.

Fitness professionals have even blended yoga into personal training and workout classes that leave students in a peaceful pool of sweat. At Noll Daniel's rigorous Urban Yoga Workout at Crunch and Apex, students do several sets of push-ups and slow, strengthening stretches, interspersed with sustained yoga positions. "Most of the strengthening comes not from the push-ups but from the yoga postures," says Daniel. "You're working against gravity, and gravity creates plenty of resistance."

Fitness guru Karen Voight likes to think of variety in exercise as akin to a variety of culinary options. "If you're tired of the same old thing, or if your favorite restaurant isn't open one night, you certainly don't go without food. You find somewhere or something else to eat." So should it be with workouts.

—*Mary Talbot*

HOW TO BEAT THE TIME CRUNCH

ARE YOU SO WEIGHED DOWN BY OBLIGATIONS THAT YOU DON'T HAVE THE TIME FOR WHAT YOU WANT TO DO? WITH THESE TIME-MANAGEMENT TIPS, YOUR LIFE CAN BE MORE FULFILLING.

My sister's idea of time management is to eat microwaved frozen dinners for weeks on end, get by with six hours of sleep a day and have her husband watch the kids when she goes off to work at the hospital at 10:00 P.M. (She works the night shift and then gets what sleep she can between 9:00 A.M. and 3:00 P.M., when her children come home from school.) She never has time to call me, so I'm the one who calls her. Our conversations go like this:

"How are you?"

"Exhausted. I had *four* hours of sleep today."

"You've got to get out of that job."

"I can't."

"Why not?"

"I don't have *time* to look for another job!"

"You've got to make time."

"I know, but I've got to go now. The kids are killing each other."

The problem with my sister is that she has been *thinking* about getting a new job with a better working schedule, and she has been *talking* about it, but she doesn't *do* anything about it—she doesn't make it her number one goal. And, according to most time-management experts, her life is unlikely to change until she commits to that goal. Unfortunately, my sister doesn't have time to hear about time management! If this sounds like you, don't panic; we've culled 24 time-management tips from several experts so that you can quickly learn some ways to put time back on your side. The first step? Take your Superwoman costume off and leave it in a phone booth.

TAKE A LOOK AT THE BIG PICTURE

"Effective time management is deciding what you really want to do in life and shifting your emphasis from doing *everything* to doing the *right* things, which will result in a sense of fulfillment and accomplishment," says Alec Mackenzie, one of the world's foremost time-management experts. Mackenzie, a management consultant, has lectured on time management to corporations in over 40 countries and written six books on the subject. Here are eight of his important theories to start you on the right track.

1. Come up with a master plan. If you don't have specific personal and professional goals in life, your dreams may not become reality. So determine your goals and, more important, commit yourself to meeting these objectives.

Your major goals should be "written down, deadlined and achievable," says Mackenzie.

2. Map it out. After charting your long-range goals, get in the habit of planning what you need and want to do in the month, week and day ahead. Write down all personal and professional events on your calendar and frequently look at the month and week ahead to get a sense of your available time and your priorities.

3. See where your time is going. You can't save time unless you know where you're wasting it. Start a time log, making detailed entries every half-hour or hour about how your day is being spent. Notations might say "7:00 A.M. to 7:20 A.M.—couldn't figure out what to wear to work" or "11:30 A.M. to 12:30 P.M.—met with my book publisher." At the end of the day "determine the priority of each action on a one-to-four scale," says Mackenzie, with one meaning very important, four meaning time was wasted.

4. Identify your time-wasters. Some of the most common time-wasters, according to Mackenzie, include indecision, lack of planning, jumping from project to project, keeping a disorganized desk, procrastinating and insisting on perfection.

5. Stay focused. List your daily goals—personal and professional—in order of priority. "Get number one finished first," says Mackenzie. "If nothing else gets done, you've checked off the most important item on the list."

6. Learn to assert yourself. If you say yes to every outside demand, you'll never get control of your time. There is, however, an art to saying no. Mackenzie recommends this four-step plan:

1. Listen—to show interest and understanding of the request.
2. Say no immediately—to avoid building up false hopes.
3. Give reasons—so the refusal will be understood.
4. Offer alternatives (if possible)—to evidence good faith.

7. Control interruptions. "It takes three times as long to recover from most interruptions as it does to endure them," says Mackenzie. Your goal should be to work on a project until it's completed; don't let the phone, mail or chatty colleagues interrupt. You can always say, "This isn't a good time for me. Can I get back to you in an hour?" Also realize that every "crisis" isn't a real crisis, says Mackenzie.

8. Build in breaks. You may be more efficient if you give yourself some breaks, even mini-breaks, throughout the day rather than always attempting to work at Concorde speed. Without fuel, Concordes crash and burn.

Now that we've looked at general time-management principles to use in the long and short term, let's zero in on how to stretch time at the office and at home.

SAVING TIME AT WORK

"Managing your time well at work means figuring out what you have to do and doing it as quickly and efficiently as possible," says J. L. Barkas, Ph.D., in her book *Creative Time Management.* Here are eight of her suggestions for working smarter, not harder.

1. Find out what your boss wants. "Rule number one for saving time at work is: Find out what is expected of you," says Dr. Barkas, and then do it.

2. Take a look at your nook. Your work environment should be thoroughly organized, whether you work in a mouse-sized cubicle or a corner office. If you don't know how to organize, go to the library for books by organizational experts. Dr. Barkas has a good rule here: "Put everything in its place. Eliminate clutter. Have readily available the tools and supplies you frequently need."

It's also a good idea to clean up your office at the end of every day so that you're not overwhelmed by the mess in the morning.

3. Streamline wherever possible. Look for ways to cut down duplicating your efforts, such as creating form letters instead of always writing an original response to every piece of correspondence. When you receive a memo requiring a short reply, handwrite that reply right onto the same memo instead of typing up an official response. Also, remember that using the phone may be even faster than writing a memo.

4. But be careful of that telephone! If compulsive talkers have your number, the telephone can be a real time trap. In general, it's best not to receive personal calls at the office: ask friends to call you *after* work. If you have an assistant, have your calls screened. An additional time-saver is to give your assistant lists of people to "always put through" or "never put through." Messages taken from the latter group should enable you to deal with their needs without engaging in lengthy phone conversations; often your assistant can call these people back with information and answers. If you don't have an assistant, Dr. Barkas suggests these four phone outs: "I have to go now"; "I can't talk much longer"; "I have someone in my office"; "I was just on my way out the door."

5. Schedule learning time. If you'll soon be switching over to a computer, "build into your work schedule the learning time that you will need to gain mastery over it—including study of the user's manual. Initially it may take more time [to do things], but in the long run, you may save time," says Dr. Barkas.

6. Delegate when you can. You don't have to be an executive to delegate, says Dr. Barkas. Delegation can mean delegating to another worker or "to a word processor or to a service such as a printing firm that will do your addressing and envelope stuffing," she adds.

7. Make meetings work. Always try to find out the purpose of a meeting so that you can attend and be prepared. If you're the one running meetings, set an agenda, start on time, end on time and don't go off on tangents. A better idea? Don't have a meeting at all if it's not really and truly *necessary*.

8. Don't panic. When you're feeling overwhelmed by a monster project, "break it down into small tasks so the work is more manageable, and set realistic deadlines," says Dr. Barkas.

SAVING TIME AT HOME

"The worst scam ever put on a woman" is the idea that she can be perfect in all spheres: a "perfect wife, unfailing mother, and flawless executive," say authors Trudi Ferguson and Joan S. Dunphy in *Answers to the Mommy Track*. So how do successful women manage these multiple, and often conflicting, roles? The authors surveyed a number of executives and came up with these time-saving (and life-saving) tips that any woman can use to balance work and personal demands.

1. Work close to home. A two-hour daily work commute adds up to a loss of 500 hours—or 21 days—a year. Consider taking a job closer to your home or even working at home.

2. Develop support systems. You shouldn't have to stay home from work because your baby-sitter has the flu. Have backup child care ready in case of emergencies. Also network with other mothers to see if you can share baby-sitting or car pooling so that you're not *always* driving Jennifer to her Saturday morning ballet class.

3. Create some routines. If chaos reigns in your household and you currently lack quality time with your family, build in predictability. For example, start a ritual of always sitting down together for dinner in the evenings— with the TV set *off*.

4. Give up complications. You don't have to attend every baby shower, serve on every committee or see "friends" you don't even like much anymore. Get your personal priorities straight: edit your calendar and address book.

5. Plan ahead now. Get your work wardrobe organized and set for the week on Sunday night. Buy ten pairs of black panty hose on sale, by catalog. Avoid grocery store lines by shopping at off-hours and stocking up. Have a filing cabinet at home where you can store important papers or passports, so you can find them when you need them.

6. Don't care what the neighbors will think. "Let go of appearances," say the authors; adopt the "if the lawn needs mowing, I don't care" approach. The world is not going to end if you don't wash the kitchen floor this week.

7. Avoid financial traps. "Take on only realistic obligations," advise the authors, so that you don't get on a treadmill. In other words, don't put yourself in the position of being stuck in a pressure-cooker job because it pays your monster Visa bills or car payments.

8. Get away from it all. All time-management experts say that vacations are essential to your overall well-being, but Dunphy and Ferguson also suggest you go away by yourself at least once every other year—even if it's only for the weekend. Use this time to recharge and rethink your personal and professional goals . . . to *dream.*

—*Kelly Good McGee*

PART NINE

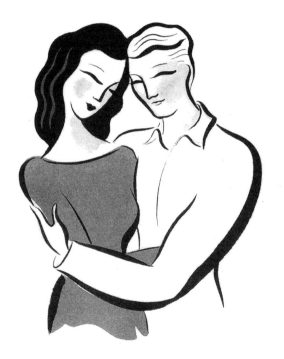

THAT SPECIAL MAN
IN YOUR LIFE

WHAT MEN CAN'T GET FROM WOMEN

ARE WE READY FOR THE MEN'S MOVEMENT, AND WHY DO THEY NEED IT ANYWAY? HERE'S A SPECIAL REPORT ON ONE OF THE MOST PROVOCATIVE TRENDS OF OUR TIME.

Twice a month, Dick Halloran, a district magistrate in Detroit, casts aside his robe, dons his blue jeans and heads off to hang out with the guys. Unlike generations of escaping males before him, however, Halloran, 43 and the father of two daughters, isn't bonding over a few rounds of golf. Instead, he and nine of his friends get together to beat on drums, chant, talk about their emotions—and even cry on one another's shoulders.

"For me, it's been spiritual," Halloran says, asserting that his wife, Bonnie, an anthropologist, also gains from his experience. "What you are doing is learning more about yourself so you can love better."

DRUMMING, SWEATING AND MASCULINE PRIDE

Welcome to the men's movement—a small-but-growing brigade of males in their thirties and forties who seek to fill the emptiness they see in their lives by turning to each other for support. Every weekend, groups gather in communities across the country, from Rogue Valley, Oregon, to New York City, to West Gardiner, Maine. Many of the meetings are small-scale, like Halloran's. Others are larger outdoor convocations that can cost from $200 to $1,500. Organizers claim the most popular events can draw up to 200 attendees, with hundreds more waiting for the chance to doff their suits, daub their faces with paint, crawl into a "sweat lodge" full of hot rocks and dance through the woods in imitation of Native American rituals.

"A man can't get deep masculine pride from a woman alone," says Marvin Allen, director of the Texas Men's Institute in San Antonio, which recently drew 700 participants to the First International Men's Conference, in Austin. Allen continues: "He gets his masculinity validated by being who he is with other men, by having them respect him and honor him for his feelings and ideas. . . . Sweating, yelling, sobbing and drumming [also] help him get it."

Not all the meetings are that frenetic, to be sure. At one drumming session I attended in New York, men spoke quietly, but with great emotion, about the lack of connection among themselves, their fathers, brothers and spouses—the same things, in fact, that women have been talking over with their friends for centuries.

Still, the discussion was not without its odd moments. "I want to be a giant to my wife," one said solemnly. The others nodded. "Ho," they said in unison, using a Native American term that the men's movement employs as a sign of affirmation.

If this sounds too bizarre to involve the nice, sensible guys you know, consider how the men's movement has seeped into popular culture. A book by the movement's leading guru—Robert Bly's *Iron John*—bestrode the best-seller list throughout 1991. The only new top-ten sitcom of the 1992 fall season, "Home Improvement," starred Tim Allen as a hapless handyman on a "quest for maleness," with a neighbor who spouts movement slogans while barbecuing squirrel in his suburban backyard. Similar storylines have figured on "Major Dad," "Cheers," "Murphy Brown" and "Coach." And even Ann Landers, that barometer of mainstream America, reports that she's now getting a thousand letters per week relating to the subject.

Why are all these men saying and doing these extraordinary things? What do they really *want*? And how can any group feel powerless when it controls the institutions of power in this country?

IN SEARCH OF A NEW MASCULINITY

The answers to these questions are almost as varied as men themselves. There's a common thread, however: the need for a new definition of masculinity to suit the nineties. As was so dramatically demonstrated during the Senate confirmation hearings for Supreme Court Justice Clarence Thomas, both sexes feel threatened these days and badly confused about how to behave.

"We've struggled with identities and relationships for the past 20 years," says Judith Langer, president of Langer Associates, a market research firm in New York that tracks lifestyle trends. Though neither men nor women want indistinguishable "unisex" roles, she says, "I don't think men are satisfied with the old-fashioned macho stuff either."

This need for a new kind of masculinity finds its strongest voice in Bly, who preaches that today's man, having grown up with a distant, workaholic father, must find the wild, free spirit within himself. The "soft" male of the seventies—epitomized by Alan Alda or Phil Donahue—won't do any longer, but neither will the raging Rambo model of the eighties.

Far from being intimidated by this, women should see that they have much to gain, Bly argues. "Women say they want you to be sensitive, but they still want you to be strong," complains Willis Reeves, 37, a special agent with the Immigration and Naturalization Service in Houston. "They don't want a wimp. How can you be sensitive and macho at the same time? We haven't figured out how to make that happen. That's why we need a movement."

Male discontent has other timely sources, too. The recession has made many question their obsession with work; if I define myself only through my job, they ask, who am I when I lose it? "Men began to see success as not all that it was cracked up to be," says Ed Poliandro, 42, a New York psychotherapist who periodically leads a men's group. Many of those discontented men are baby boomers who are now hitting middle age—and as usual, what bothers the boomers reverberates throughout society. Or as Sidney Siller, founder of the National Organization for Men, puts it, "There's a lot of angst out there."

There's a lot of hankering for the olden days, too, at least as we imagine them. Just as some women dream about jam-making and quilting like Great-Grandma, some men want to be out there hunting buffalo like Kevin Costner.

Bly, 64, who won the National Book Award for poetry in 1968, doesn't deny the mythological element of the movement he started: In fact, his prose best-seller, *Iron John*, is named after a hairy fairy-tale character.

Himself the father of five, Bly declares that men need the mentors of maleness they had in preindustrial times, when fathers taught their sons their trade. To try to foster that kind of togetherness, he began holding "gatherings of men" ten years ago in northern California and New Mexico. But it took a Bill Moyers documentary about him, aired on PBS in 1990, to make him a household name; since then, his book has sold more than 500,000 copies, and he now commands several thousand dollars for a single appearance at a weekend gathering.

CRITICS ABOUND

Every man doesn't buy Bly's message, to be sure. The movement remains heavily white, white-collar and middle-class, as even adherents admit. And Native Americans have a few problems with the movement's appropriation of their symbols.

Feminists are troubled as well by many aspects of this movement, not least the argument that it's patterned after their own. "I really resent analogies of it to the women's movement," says pioneering feminist and author Betty Friedan. "The men's movement is preaching a definition of masculinity based on dominance in false caveman's clothes."

Bly shrugs off such criticism. "If people don't get angry at what you're saying, you're not saying anything. Betty Friedan seems very threatened by the whole thing, partly because it doesn't fit any of the old feminist categories."

Yet he also allows that the women's movement has "been wonderful in looking at the truth of the pain women have been in for a long time. Society tells men, 'I don't think it's right to express pain.' All the truth-telling is to the good."

But *are* these men really telling—and facing—the truth? Some critics contend that they're actually reverting to adolescence and refusing to deal with problems of family and intimacy. By emphasizing their distance from women, these critics say, the men's movement is polarizing the sexes even further. "They're taking unreal postures of adolescence and making them tolerable," says William Simon, Ph.D., a sociology professor at the University of Houston. "The movement is robbing us of an opportunity to bring men and women closer together."

"Bly's route is wrong," adds Michael Kimmel, Ph.D., a sociology professor at the State University of New York at Stony Brook and spokesperson for the National Organization for Men against Sexism. "I believe the men's feelings are real, but it's dishonest to say it has nothing to do with feminism and that the separation is not in some way running away from women. How will going off in the woods, ripping off my shirt and barking animal noises make me a more caring lover? How will it make me a better father?"

Experts aren't the only ones who take this view. Willis Reeves, while willing to admit that men should get in touch with their feelings, isn't quite ready for all-out primitivism. "Stripping naked and getting into a sauna?" he says doubtfully. "I have problems with that."

Bob Stem, a high school football coach from Easton, Pennsylvania, has an even more basic dispute: He believes that men would do better to devote less time to crying over their relationships with their fathers—and more to being with their *own* kids. "It's a cop-out," he says curtly. "People don't spend enough time with their kids."

Most serious, however, is the criticism that the men's movement, by focusing on raw emotion and power, may indirectly contribute to the current wave of violence against women.

Says Susan Faludi, author of *Backlash: The Undeclared War against American Women*, "The men's movement is not to blame for the rise in sexual violence. But it's certainly running on a parallel track with other manifestations of men's rage over what is perceived as women's growing power."

NURTURING A NEW MOVEMENT

Defenders say the movement can offer a legitimate, healthy outlet for those emotions. "The whole violence issue is one that the men leading retreats need to take on," says Forrest Craver, a leader of men's retreats from Washington, D.C. And even Eleanor Smeal, president of the Feminist Majority Foundation, says cautiously, "I hope the men's movement would lead to a society that would put down male violence."

Many plead for the movement to be given time, noting that a certain amount of overkill is almost inevitable in any kind of risk-taking—even, perhaps, in the early days of consciousness-raising among women.

Says Chris Harding, editor of a movement magazine called *Wingspan: Journal of the Male Spirit,* "Women need to be patient with men involved in the movement. It's like a man supporting a woman in her career or pursuing a degree."

There are signs that women are willing to exhibit that patience, at least for the time being. According to Bly's editor, William Patrick, they now constitute a substantial percentage of the book's purchasers. In any case, after having complained for so long that men never talk about their emotions, some women wonder whether they dare rebuff them now. Consider the words of history professor John Guarnaschelli, 51, who's been married for 26 years and organizes meetings in New York. "I didn't realize I had feelings besides love and sex feelings," he says. "I've learned to be more intimate with myself, and as a result, I've been more intimate with my wife."

Or listen to Bonnie, Dick Halloran's wife of 19 years, who says she wasn't crazy about his meetings with the boys in the beginning but has come to appreciate them. "He's a happier, fuller person and brings strength to our relationship." She pauses. "The drumming is something I wouldn't do, but why should I deny someone an experience they find meaningful?"

As they say around the campfire, "Ho."

— *Tom Lowry*

PRIVATE WARS
OF LOVING COUPLES

COMPETITION BETWEEN SPOUSES IS NORMAL AND
CAN EVEN BE GOOD FOR A MARRIAGE. BUT
ALWAYS TRYING TO ONE-UP EACH OTHER CAN
MEAN YOU'RE HEADED FOR TROUBLE.

Competition is a basic fact of life. Most of us consider it normal on the job, at school and, of course, in sports. But the idea of married people competing with each other seems ugly. The fact is, though, that in many marriages, at some point both husband and wife may become aware of envy and one-upmanship. Even couples who pride themselves on being equals may wonder, "Is there *really* room in this relationship for two successful people? Or if one of us advances, is the other one diminished?"

One couple I counseled, for instance, decided together that it was important for the wife to stay home for at least a year after their first child was born. She loved her job but said she was willing to make the sacrifice. Her husband was happy with the arrangement as long as she seemed to be comfortable with it.

At first the wife did enjoy staying home with the baby, and she loved listening to her husband describe the exciting details of his workday. But after about six months at home, she began to feel as if she were on the sidelines while he'd become the star. It became increasingly difficult for her to curb her resentment and be enthusiastic about his growing success.

HEADING FOR A CRISIS

One activity this couple had always enjoyed together was playing doubles tennis with their friends. They'd been a great, cooperative team, but now the wife started criticizing her husband's game. Before they knew it, they'd become fiercely competitive, and one day she instigated a vicious argument over a missed shot. Both of them were quite alarmed by this, and they decided to consult with me.

In our session the wife started by describing the tennis-court squabble. I asked her what was happening in the marriage, beyond the tennis court. The wife then pinpointed the real issue: the fact that her husband's career was moving full steam ahead while hers was on hold. Finally she said, "I feel just awful saying this, but I'm insanely jealous of my own husband!"

I'm finding competitiveness as a marital theme more common these days, so I decided to bring a few couples together to discuss their experiences. In addition to this couple, the group included a pair of teachers; the husband felt competitive with the wife because she'd been made chairman of her department and was earning more than he was. Like the first couple, these partners competed about certain issues. The third couple, both deeply involved in community theater, were extremely competitive—virtually every area of their lives seemed fair game for one-upping each other.

FERRETING OUT THE HIDDEN AGENDA

Spouses compete with each other on many levels: A wife who feels uncomfortable when her husband prepares dinner may feel that only she knows what's right for the family; a husband may put down his wife's friends. In both scenarios one partner tries to feel better about himself or herself by getting the edge on the spouse. Frequently, though, a spouse may be denying his or her competitive feelings.

For example, the wife who was jealous of her husband's career was too uncomfortable with the competitive side of her nature to admit to her husband—or to herself—how she really felt. Rather than address her feelings, she pushed them out of her mind. But instead her true feelings got played out on the tennis court.

Competition in marriage doesn't have to be a negative experience, one involving outdoing your partner. When your husband's good at something, you may be inspired to live up to his example, not necessarily to surpass him. For example, if he's calm and in charge when your child has a temper tantrum, you may think, "If he can do it, so can I!" It's not that you want to do a better job than he's doing—you just want to be the best parent you can be.

Competitive feelings are normal and can keep you and your mate on your toes, giving each of you a healthy way to measure your behavior and accomplishments. In a symmetrical relationship, spouses see each other as soul mates and partners. They believe they can learn from and support each other. One partner may be having more success attaining a goal than the other, but it's understood that at a different time the positions may be reversed.

Still, marital competitiveness should be monitored. Sometimes another dynamic kicks in and competitiveness spirals. Then, without being completely conscious of it, the couple jostles for power, domination and control. They try to one-up each other to make themselves feel good, and so undercut each other's self-esteem with subtle put-downs.

This was the pattern followed by the intensely competitive couple. When the husband was made chairman of fund-raising for a local theater group, his wife became head of its renovation committee. Each spouse then tried to get the edge on the other. Whenever the husband gave reports at monthly meetings, he'd steal his wife's thunder by making her announcements for her.

This couple often seemed as if they were trying to squash each other. The husband would say such things as "My wife doesn't take risks the way I do" or "I'm a better cook." The wife, feeling criticized and put down, would respond, "He doesn't know anything about dealing with the kids."

This husband and wife had started seeing each other only as standards by which to measure themselves. Instead of judging each other on their individual strengths and talents, they had set up criteria that doomed the other to fail. For them, the more one person failed, the more the other succeeded.

There's another fascinating dynamic I'd like to point out. I still see many, many women deliberately play down a one-up position in order to protect their husband from feeling one-down. This is exactly what happened in the case of the teaching couple. The wife began to minimize her promotion and pay raise to protect her husband's ego. But despite her downplaying, her husband started to feel as if he'd lost his edge. One night he jokingly asked his wife, "Do you think I'm a better-looking man than you are a woman?"

The wife didn't find it funny; in fact, she was dismayed by his remark. "Before then I'd never quite realized how competitive we'd become," she told the group.

DEALING WITH COMPETITION

Let's start with the woman who was jealous of her husband's career. In a healthy way her own competitive feelings toward her husband were motivating her to act. Those feelings made her face facts. She was no longer fulfilled staying home, and her career was in danger of being short-circuited. Once she decided to return to work, she and her husband sat down and talked about the next stage. He not only supported her decision but also pitched in by researching daycare options.

In the case of the teachers, the husband made a move, too. Instead of being eaten alive by his competitive feelings toward his wife, he decided to go to graduate school for his master's in special education—a goal he'd previously put aside. As his chafing sense of being one-down to his wife eased, she no longer had to put herself down to salve his ego.

But when a couple keep tearing each other down instead of spurring each other on, they have to take careful stock of their behavior. When the third, very competitive couple did this, something finally clicked with the husband. He realized that rather than judge his achievements on their own merits, the only way he'd been able to feel successful was to stay one step ahead of his wife's accomplishments.

Once he'd looked at it this way, he came to see that his competitiveness stemmed from his childhood experience, which is not uncommon. Back then, though it had always been done in a seemingly fun-loving way, beneath the surface he and his brothers had been jockeying for the position of Daddy's favorite son. In a way, he was still trying for that.

Like these couples, you can learn to keep competition in check. If you can feel terrific about yourself only by judging your mate and knocking him down, make a conscious decision to shift your focus and take a look at what in your own life you could improve. Avoid internalizing intense competitive feelings. Talk them out with your spouse so you can defuse a potentially explosive situation.

At the end of our sessions, each couple could clearly see just how the competitive dimension operated in their particular relationship. The wife who'd been jealous of her husband had to laugh at herself when she recalled the day they first met. They had been on a ski slope and had not yet been formally introduced. The first thing he'd done was take the lead down the mountain; next she'd led him to a steeper slope. All afternoon they took turns pushing each other a little further.

"I loved the challenge as much as he did," she said. "And I loved that we were gentle with each other at the same time." This day set the tone for their marriage: one that challenges and stimulates *both* partners to do and be their very best.

—*Sonya Rhodes*

IS YOUR HUSBAND SEXUALLY INSECURE?

IT'S EVERY MAN'S DEEPEST SECRET: HIS FEAR THAT HE'S NOT A GOOD LOVER. HE WON'T TALK ABOUT IT, BUT YOU CAN HELP PUT SEXUAL ANXIETY TO REST.

When her husband's sex drive took a nosedive, Julia suspected that Joe, 36, was having an affair. "We'd been married five years and never had any problems in bed before," says Julia, 31. "But then we started having sex less and less—it was down to about once a month, and only when I initiated it. When we did make love, it felt awkward, like he wasn't really enjoying it. The only explanation I could come up with was that he was getting sex somewhere else. But when I confronted him about it, he insisted nothing was wrong."

In fact, Joe wasn't having an affair—he was just as worried about their sex life as Julia was. "It started one night when I couldn't get hard. Julia was understanding, but I was freaked—it had never happened to me before, and all I could think about was that it might happen again, then that I'd never get another erection. And if I couldn't please her, she'd have an affair, or leave me. Every time I thought about having sex, the anxiety got worse."

Joe's problem, say sex therapists, strikes most men at some point in their lives. It's called sexual insecurity—the feeling that you just don't measure up in bed. And in men, impotence—the inability to get or sustain an erection—isn't the only trigger. "Male sexual insecurity is caused by anything that makes a man feel unimportant, undesirable, not quite adequate," says psychologist Bernie Zilbergeld, Ph.D., author of *The New Male Sexuality.* "Sex is just like sports—people don't perform well when their self-esteem is low."

The number of men showing signs of sexual insecurity is rising, experts say, and one reason is a new kind of tension caused by shifts in our sex roles. "Masculinity is being redefined—it used to be all about power and aggression. Now men are expected to be emotional and nurturing and to share in traditionally female tasks like raising children," says Shirley Zussman, Ed.D., a Manhattan-based sex and marital therapist. Even though men are striving to adjust to less macho standards outside the bedroom, the belief that sexual prowess is the ultimate proof of manhood persists. In a recent Roper poll of 1,000 men, two out of three said men ought to be more caring and sensitive. But when asked which qualities they associate with "practically all men," the top answer was "having a strong sex drive." "Being able to show emotions" came in last.

"Men's idea of what it means to be masculine is still tied up in their sexuality," says Dr. Zussman.

A TABOO TOPIC

The knowledge that many men feel anxious in bed may come as a surprise, since most men won't admit they're feeling sexually insecure. "Men don't talk about it because the belief persists that a man should always be ready, willing and able to have sex—no matter what," says Dr. Zussman. If he's not, there must be something wrong with him: He's a wimp. "It's much more acceptable for a woman to be unsure of her lovemaking skills or insecure about her body," she says. "But many men have the same fears as women—they just show up in different ways."

Just like the teenager who mopes around until you ask, "What's wrong?" the sexually insecure man is probably sending you plenty of silent signals. "His lovemaking may seem mechanical, like he's not really involved. That's a sign that he can't let himself go, because he's too caught up in worrying about whether he's pleasing his partner," says Dr. Zussman. "He may be reluctant to try anything new in bed, because he feels safer following the same script every time, or he may avoid sex." Some men withdraw from any physical affection. "Hugging and kissing his partner might make her think he wants to make love, and that makes him anxious," says Dr. Zussman.

A man may make excuses for his lack of sexual enthusiasm—saying he's tired or not in the mood—but it's also common for him to lash out at his partner. Connor, 34, hasn't been interested in sex lately, and he thinks he knows why: "Laurie, my wife, has no regard for my mood. She'll tickle me, or start giggling, when I want her to take sex seriously. So I get defensive and start mentally listing her faults instead of making love to her." Usually, he says, rather than talk to her about it, he loses his desire and just goes to sleep. Says Dr. Zussman, "It's easier for a man to blame his wife for not being sexy or loving enough to arouse him than to admit he's insecure."

HER SEXUAL PAST

The pressure men feel to measure up sexually is higher than ever before, thanks to widespread social changes. Few women these days are virgins when they marry, and their expectations of lovemaking have risen along with their experience. Women are now more likely than men to want to introduce new sexual activities to lovemaking, notes New York psychiatrist and sex therapist Avodah Offit, M.D. A woman's sexual knowledge and curiosity can be exciting to her partner, but it can also make him insecure. Although a husband may enjoy his wife's assertiveness in bed, he's still conditioned to believe it's his job to be the sex teacher, initiator and experimenter. "When a woman takes charge, it can make him feel less like a man, especially if she is *too* aggressive or demanding," says Dr. Offit.

"It took me a long time to get used to Jill's sexual proficiency," says Paul, 33. "She knows exactly what to do in order to come. It really put me off at first—it seemed so mechanical, so professional. She would make it clear that she wanted oral sex, and I'd perform it, but there was no joy in it for me. I felt like a masturbation device."

Insecure men may also interpret a woman's eagerness to experiment as subtle criticism of their lovemaking. "A wife may say, 'I want you to *really* make love to me,'" says Dr. Offit. "To her husband, that sounds like a challenge, making him feel like his performance is going to be judged and increasing his anxiety."

But it's not just a woman's sexual knowledge that feeds men's insecurity—it's also the fear that she may be comparing him to past lovers. "Men are conditioned to compete with each other, especially sexually, so even the mention of an old boyfriend can make a guy feel inadequate," says Dr. Zilbergeld. Peter, 24, thinks his wife, Peggy, is finding fault with him whenever she talks about an ex-lover. "It's as though she's mentally comparing me to him. She must think I'm lacking something, otherwise why would she bring him up?"

FROM SUCCESS OBJECT TO SEX OBJECT

The newest trend in advertising is the use of sexy male bodies to sell products, says Judith Langer, president of Langer Associates, a market research firm in New York—and it's making many men feel insecure about their physical attractiveness. "Everywhere you look you see pictures of very attractive men oozing sensuality, like in the Calvin Klein ads, and it's putting pressure on men to measure up. It used to be enough for a man to be rich and powerful. Now he has to be rich, powerful *and* a hunk," says Langer.

It's no surprise to experts that idealized images of male attractiveness have a negative influence on men. "Women's bodies have been used in ads for a long time, with the result that women are always comparing themselves to these unrealistic standards," says Ann Kearney-Cooke, Ph.D., a psychologist in Cincinnati who specializes in body image and eating disorders. "Now men are starting to do that, too, and are suffering the same loss of self-esteem."

In fact, in a recent survey of 2,000 people conducted with Ruth Striegel-Moore, Ph.D., assistant professor of psychology at Wesleyan University in Middletown, Connecticut, Dr. Kearney-Cooke found that men were as self-conscious about their bodies as women and rated the importance of their own attractiveness equally high.

The prevalence of male nudity in popular culture also encourages women to be more open about their appreciation of men's bodies, and men are getting the message. "Women are being given permission to ogle these men, and their partners can't help but notice. It makes them feel less desirable, less sure of themselves as sexual partners," says Dr. Zussman.

THE BIG "O"

All men want to be great lovers, but the criteria have changed. There was a time when a man graded his sexual performance on how good *he* felt. Now he often grades it by how fast or how often he can make *her* have an orgasm. If she takes a long time or doesn't climax at all, he worries that he's a rotten lover.

Tony, 29, says that it takes two hours for his wife to have an orgasm. The other 22 hours of the day he's deeply in love with Anita, but he dreads having sex with her. "It's too much work," he says. He's still aroused by her—but he avoids sex and the anxiety it causes. Asked why he doesn't talk to Anita about it or give up on her orgasm, he answers that he doesn't want to be "a pig," that she's entitled to climax. "I'd rather skip sex than not give her an orgasm."

This puts pressure on women, too. Says Anne, 41, "I've finally gotten Bill to stop asking, 'Did you come?' But I know he's still obsessed with my orgasm. If I don't climax, he's going to feel bad. So I either have an orgasm, fake one or don't have one and feel bad that he's feeling bad. It's hard to relax enough to climax."

THE DUAL-CAREER DILEMMA

The fastest-growing sexual complaint among women is "loss of interest in sex due to the pressures of working and raising children," says Dr. Zilbergeld. Unfortunately, men are apt to take it personally. Tim, 38, says that his wife, Karen, 37, is preoccupied with her teaching job and their two children. He'll initiate lovemaking, he says, but if he gets the idea that her mind is on other matters, he'll swiftly lose interest. "Sometimes it seems like she's not even there, and I might as well be masturbating," he says. "Sex is supposed to be interactive, a way to show affection and involvement. When she's unresponsive, it feels like I'm not important to her. It hurts my feelings."

Karen responds, "It's unrealistic of him to expect me to come home from a rough day, take care of the kids, then leap into bed and be ready to go. I know that if he's patient, I'll come around. But he says he needs proof of my involvement right away, otherwise he loses his interest."

THE AGE GAP

Unlike women, who peak sexually in their thirties or later, men in their thirties are starting to see their sexual powers decline. For example, the average time it takes for a 40-year-old man to get another erection after orgasm is 20 to 30 minutes, compared with only 10 minutes or less when he was 20. Most men also need more physical stimulation as they age—they can't get hard just from looking at sexy pictures or having fantasies. No man brushes these changes off lightly, says Dr. Zussman, and even men who have no trouble getting or keeping an erection are sensitive to any reminder of aging. "I've started to round out a little, and I hate it when my wife pats my tummy," says Terry, 42. "So far, I'm performing fine sexually, but the other physical changes are the handwriting on the wall. Some day, inevitably, my hard-ons will vanish, my teeth will fall out—I don't like to think about that."

BOOSTING SEXUAL CONFIDENCE

The first step toward relieving sexual insecurity, say experts, is communication. But how do you broach the subject without making a man feel even more insecure? "Never talk about a sexual problem during sex—that only provokes more anxiety. Bring it up in a supportive atmosphere, when both of you are in good moods," says Dr. Zilbergeld. "Try not to be accusatory. Avoid closing in for the kill by saying, 'You always go limp when . . . .' Instead, you could tell him, 'This is my impression.' Most men will respond well to this kind of discussion."

The good news is that if a man has no underlying physical problems, "his sexual functioning generally improves when his anxiety is reduced," says Helen Singer Kaplan, M.D., Ph.D., director of the Human Sexuality Program at the New York Hospital—Cornell Medical Center in New York City. Moreover, the same cultural changes that have heightened men's sexual insecurity may also make it easier for them to talk openly about it and, as a result, feel more confident. Says Joe, who worried that his wife might leave him if he couldn't perform, "Talking about our sex life made me realize I'd been attributing thoughts and expectations to Julia that she wasn't even feeling. That took away my anxiety and made us a team again."

Experts say it's common for men to approach sex like a contest they have to "win," putting added pressure on themselves to perform. If sex isn't going well one night, give your husband, and yourself, permission to stop: Suggest calling it quits and just hold each other or talk. Reminding him there's always another time will help him feel more secure.

"Many couples are starting to understand that great sex isn't about performance," says Dr. Kearney-Cooke. "It's about being honest with your partner and letting yourself be vulnerable. That's a lot more difficult—and ultimately more rewarding."

—Kate Nolan

FRANK ANSWERS TO 22 SEX QUESTIONS

EVERY KID HAS QUESTIONS ABOUT SEX,
AND MOST NEVER DO GET GOOD ANSWERS.
HERE ARE SOME ANSWERS, FOR ADULTS,
FROM A NOTED SEX THERAPIST.

A woman's capacity for sexual fulfillment does not necessarily protect her from sexual embarrassment. She may have splendid orgasms, yet she may be unable to direct her lover to help her reach them. She may be capable of a wide range of erotic fantasy yet be ashamed to enjoy it. Or she may be capable of making passionate love yet still allow herself to settle for monotony.

The sources of embarrassment are sometimes complex, rooted so deeply in a person's psyche that they can't be pinpointed. Yet frequently a simple, direct solution works to encourage a breakthrough.

The following questions about sex are derived from my experience in private practice. They cover a variety of the most universal problems. And they are all directed toward the relief of intimate pain. Rarely are any remedies an absolute panacea for the distresses of body or soul. Yet even simple questions and answers can provide an enlightening step toward the discovery of our sexual selves.

Q: **1. I need to be caressed all over before intercourse. My lover has recently begun to proceed directly to my genitals. He doesn't seem to hear me telling him what I need.**

A: Being direct and specific is best. Say, for example, "I need at least 15 minutes of general caressing before you touch my breasts or my clitoris." Be prepared to repeat the request.

Q: **2. I climax quickly by myself. When my lover stimulates me, I take much longer to have an orgasm, and sometimes I don't come at all. What's wrong with me?**

A: Nothing. You're simply used to your own method of stimulation. He can't read your mind. When you're comfortable enough to tell and show him exactly what you want, you'll begin to enjoy better results. But don't be disappointed if your lover's method of stimulating you differs from your own: Some men can't master the small-muscle finger movements necessary to stimulate a woman's clitoris. I call this condition sexual dyskinesia. Your lover's ability may increase with patient guidance, but it can happen very slowly or not at all.

Q: **3. My partner wants to have intercourse every day, while I'm happy doing it just once or twice a week. I'd hate to lose him because of mismatched libidos.**

A: I'd suggest that the two of you plan to have sex once or twice a week at specific times. This might alleviate his anxiety and reassure him of your basic interest in him as a lover. Even though this may seem mechanical, removing the element of uncertainty surrounding your sexual activity may simultaneously reduce his need and increase your own desire to be a more spontaneous partner.

Q: **4. How do you ask for oral sex? I can't have an orgasm without it, so I'm often left frustrated, but I worry that there's a reason some men are so reluctant to do this.**

A: If you have intimate physical sex, you are certainly close enough to ask an intimate question, like: How do you feel about oral sex? Your partner may or may not confess distaste. In general, though, unless you are aware of a strong odor on yourself (which could be a sign of infection and should be checked out), chances are good that your partner is experiencing psychological inhibition. You might try to gently explore the matter further with him, or reassure him when he does perform oral sex that you're enjoying yourself. Many men are unsure about exactly how to give a woman pleasure in that way and choose not to simply because they're afraid of being inadequate lovers.

Q: **5. I've recently been fantasizing about other men (besides my lover) during sex. How can I stop my thoughts?**

A: Attempts at thought control during sex can only prohibit pleasure. Don't underestimate fantasy—imagination is a powerful aphrodisiac. However, if sex is physically unpleasant or you're hostile to your partner, you should try to improve reality rather than hide in your fantasy.

Q: **6. I tire during sex because my lover needs up to an hour to ejaculate. How can I last longer?**

A: Tell him to stop when you get tired. He can ejaculate later.

Q: **7. I've never climaxed during intercourse, but my lover always asks me if I've "come." Is it wrong for me to fake contractions and tell him that he's great?**

A: Faking orgasm may prevent you from ever enjoying a real one. Better to admire your partner's patience than to flatter his sexual prowess.

Q: **8. My partner enjoys anal sex, although I don't much like it. What should I do?**

A: If the activity causes both of you no pain or infection, I see occasional indulgence as an expression of monogamous love. However, if anal sex is an exclusive fetish or an overwhelming preoccupation—or either of you gets urinary tract infections despite precautions—the issue requires unequivocal resolution.

Q: **9. I refuse to perform fellatio, but my partner feels his life is barren and incomplete without it. Is there any hope for our sex life?**

A: In the past, men found or hired other women to gratify their desire for oral sex. These days, it's better for the two of you to try to reach some kind of compromise. If you can't, a long-term relationship might be difficult unless you bond so strongly that it compensates for chronic sexual dissatisfaction.

Q: **10. Though my lover ejaculates rapidly, he has a strong second erection soon after. Should he use it or learn to last longer the first time?**

A: Both! Most women prefer a longer first intercourse, and most men enjoy that first ejaculation more if they last longer. But some women find that intercourse after ejaculation is the ultimate well-lubricated excitement. Each person deserves a choice of the best.

Q: **11. What does it say about me if the only men with whom I enjoy having sex are either married or committed?**

A: Since you can't marry a married man, you may have an unconscious desire to remain an unmarried child. You may also have an unresolved Oedipal complex, a need to compete with the mother (the other woman) in order to win the father. Obviously, having a productive relationship with a man of your own would be simpler if he didn't belong to someone else first.

Q: **12. My lover enjoys sex only if I wear spike-heeled boots and leather underwear and order him to perform sexual services. Frankly, it's become a boring game. What should I do?**

A: Your lover wants you to be a dominatrix, to excite him by control, humiliation or even pain. Psychotherapy might help him—or it might not. You may want to reconsider the relationship.

Q: **13. I often think about having sex with two men at the same time. Is that perverse?**

A: Although erotic fantasies generally contain perverse elements, having such fantasies is not considered aberrant unless they interfere with daily life or spark destructive behavior.

Q: **14. I'm in love with a man who has premature ejaculation. I plan to marry him anyway, but can he ever be totally cured?**

A: Many virile young men ejaculate quickly because that is nature's most efficient guarantee of insemination. You can't "cure" a natural bodily function. But virtually all men can learn to delay ejaculation with techniques that increase awareness and, if necessary, help to reduce abnormal anxiety.

Q: **15. I feel very sexual when I'm flirting and kissing, but I don't enjoy actual genital contact. I can't tell whether my problem is physical or psychological.**

A: It's probably psychological. Something in your past could have turned you off to sexual touching and closeness. However, if you are experiencing actual pain when you are touched, you should investigate a physical cause.

Q: **16. A man I'm dating admits his homosexual past. He's healthy and wants to be heterosexual from now on. Should I trust him?**

A: Some homosexuals can't be aroused enough by a woman to get an erection; others can experience a reflex erection without erotic feeling. True bisexuals are attracted to both women and men. Try having an open talk with him; it may help you develop realistic expectations about the relationship. As for trust, honesty and homosexuality are independent traits.

Q: **17. Is it really possible to continue a friendship with a man after you've stopped having sex?**

A: That depends on why the sexual relationship stopped. If you've been cruelly rejected, continuing a friendship would be masochistic. However, when sexual relations cease by mutual consent, friendship seems an appropriate sequel.

Q: **18. I've adopted celibacy to protect myself against AIDS—I refuse to suffer STD anxiety. Will I have sex problems when I get married?**

A: I can't predict. If you're totally avoiding sex, you're more likely to be inhibited than self-protective. And remember that marriage alone doesn't necessarily protect you from AIDS.

Q: **19. How can I feel comfortable if my partner won't wear a condom?**

A: You can't. You shouldn't. Unless you're certain beyond a reasonable doubt of your partner's health and fidelity, you must insist on a condom. Your discomfort seems to reflect a lurking suspicion; you don't seem sure enough of him to allow him to dispense with protection.

Q: **20. I recently had a lesbian relationship that ended when I found my lover needed more attention than I could give. Now I'm attracted to a man who wants only to take care of me. Am I bisexual, gay, heterosexual or just fickle?**

A: Your attractions seem based more on dependency needs than on sexuality. You should consider which gender you most enjoy erotically. Then you can select an appropriate partner for the exchange of sex and other dependencies.

Q: **21. I'm afraid to lose a friendship with a male friend by having an affair with him. Is this loss inevitable?**

A: Sex tests friendship. But if the connection has value, it will survive the intensity—and demise—of physical passion. Indeed, some of the best friendships I know of exist between former lovers who discontinued their affairs for practical reasons.

Q: **22. My lover says that my intellect is his major erotic attraction. Wouldn't it be better if he were mainly attracted to my body?**

A: Many people have found intellectual attraction to be the key to a lasting erotic relationship. The freshness of a woman's mind can be a crucial element in sustaining a man's sexual interest. Besides which, simple physical attraction is rarely eternal.

— *Avodah K. Offit, M.D.*

PART TEN

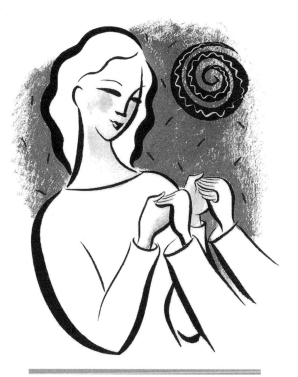

NURTURING YOUR
RELATIONSHIPS

THE INCREDIBLE HEALING POWER OF FAMILY RITUALS

IN A SOCIETY THAT'S LOSING ITS GRIP ON WHAT'S IMPORTANT, RITUALS HELP COUPLES AND KIDS AFFIRM WHAT THEY MEAN TO ONE ANOTHER.

Rituals?" said my friend Debby when I asked if she and her husband had any. "Gee, I don't know . . . ." She sounded dubious but promised she would think about it. Two hours later my phone rang; it was Debby, seeming more hopeful. "I thought of one: I do the vacuuming, but Frank changes the bag. Does that count?"

Well, no, it didn't, I told her, though at this point part of me wished it did. I'd asked about 20 of my friends and acquaintances, all married, all parents, the same question. Most drew blanks when it came to husband-and-wife rituals. Everyone had rituals that involved the kids—birthdays, of course, and holiday celebrations—but we all felt we were anemic here, too. The psychologists and anthropologists who study rituals had given me a few simple ingredients: a ritual, unlike a habit or a chore, has a symbolic content that provides meaning for the people involved; it gets repeated with some regularity; and, as one expert put it, "If it doesn't happen, someone knows it." Sex didn't count.

I should have known I'd get myself into trouble by mentioning that last qualifier. "Who has time for sex?" was the usual remark, give or take a few guffaws. And the best my friends could come up with, when I asked about rituals, were ways of dividing labor: "He drives, I'm the navigator"; "I cook, the kids clean up." My question had a demoralizing effect. "We should have more, I know, but . . . ," everyone said, sounding as if they had just flunked something.

"There *are* fewer rituals today," says Jerome Kagan, Ph.D., a professor of psychology at Harvard University. "It's one of the crises of modern life," particularly poignant because "humans by their very nature demand something transcendental about their lives. We get depressed if we just eat and sleep and do our work," he explains.

If rituals are a good thing—adding texture to life—why are we settling for farina?

HOW RITUALS WORK THEIR MAGIC

Studies confirm that rituals are on the decline, particularly eating dinner together, the most basic of rites, considered the barometer of a family's stability. It's a victim of two-career couples, single-parent households and overcommitted lives. A survey of 400 families in Seattle found that in 55 percent of the families who did eat dinner together, the meal actually lasted only 20 minutes or less—a kind of communal eat-and-run. And rituals shared with an extended family—Sunday afternoon spent with cousins or with grandparents, for example—exist for many of us only in Norman Rockwell paintings.

While no one contends that rituals can make or break a family, it's clear they have incredible power as balm and ballast in even the most emotionally fragile families. In fact, recent studies of alcoholic families show that children whose families have managed to maintain some rituals—family dinners, regular bedtime routines, celebrations—are less likely to become alcoholics or marry alcoholics. Steven Wolin, M.D., a clinical professor of psychiatry and behavioral science at the Family Research Center at George Washington University in Washington, D.C., has co-conducted several such studies with Linda Bennett, Ph.D., a professor of anthropology at Memphis State University in Tennessee. Dr. Wolin, author of *The Resilient Self: How Survivors of Troubled Families Rise above Adversity*, says these conclusions apply to families troubled in other ways as well—by divorce, a parent's mental illness or the dispiriting effects of poverty. "Rituals can be protective, even in families with severe problems," he explains.

Indeed, research strongly suggests rituals are not only a reflection of a family's stability but a vital contributor to it, says Barbara Fiese, Ph.D., an assistant professor of psychology at Syracuse University in New York.

Family rituals—dinnertime, storytime, weekend outings, annual vacations, rites of passage (birthdays, graduations)—"allow children to come up with an identity in the family and outside of it," says Dr. Fiese, "to experience feelings of belonging," and to know the significance of both continuity and change in life.

STRANGERS IN THE NIGHT

Most people I know feel their family ritual life is less rich than it should be—but their couple ritual life is practically nonexistent.

My friends and I did recollect, however, that the early days of our marriages were much different. Alice and her husband used to do something they called "gazing": They would lie in bed before going to sleep every night and just . . . look at each other. John told me about the late-night bike rides he and his wife used to take—just the two of them flying along. Debby used to walk her husband partway to the office every morning. Other friends recalled languid Sunday mornings in bed with the newspaper, reading aloud to each other; the weekly never-missed, campy nighttime soap opera—"Dallas" or "Dynasty"—watched with two spoons and a pint of Ben and Jerry's Heath Bar Crunch. We all sounded as if we were describing different people. "A couple in its initial phase establishes its identity through ritual," Dr. Wolin says. My friends and I had given up all these rituals somewhere along the way; we'd established an identity—only to lose it.

One reason we have difficulty seeing rituals in our life is we're stuck with outmoded fifties' and early sixties' notions of what they should be, says Dr. Fiese. "If our ideas about rituals are different from those of our childhood, we feel we aren't doing it right," adds Helen Fisher, Ph.D., a research associate in anthropology at the American Museum of Natural History in New York City and author of *Anatomy of Love*. "Time is so dramatically changing the American couple and family that traditional rituals are breaking down. We're creating new rituals, but we don't call them that because they don't tie the past to the present."

The first step to embracing more rituals in your life is noticing the untraditional ones you may already have. My friend Betsy, who is the mother of two young children, said almost as an afterthought that her husband makes her coffee every morning. He grinds the beans (from a special blend he buys), brews the coffee and pours it into a treasured mug. It was very clear, once she began telling me about it, that this lovingly prepared cup of coffee is very important to both of them—she loves it and he loves doing it. Every Sunday my sister and her husband, who have three children under age seven, separately read the "Personality Parade" column in their newspaper supplement and then, after the kids are in bed, quiz each other on the movie-star minutiae in it—cracking each other up in the process.

There's a point to looking again at the rituals we've already got: If we think about them, we'll appreciate them more and be eager to create others.

GETTING BACK TO BASICS

Somehow, though, this talk about the rituals we *do* have, while heartening, doesn't go far enough. I sense that most of my friends still feel their ritual life is skimpy. Indeed, family therapists Janine Roberts, Ed.D., and Evan Imber-Black, Ph.D., coauthors of *Rituals for Our Times*, are "struck by how much people want to return to rituals—to evoke their values in new ways." But most are at a loss as to how to do so. Other family therapists suggest tried-and-true rituals—with a twist—to help fill in that gap. For example, it's not that the dinner hour holds some magical ingredient for family bliss, but that sitting at a table for a set period during which people talk about what's on their minds is powerful medicine.

So if your family is unable to meet daily at sundown, get together at breakfast to talk, or schedule two unbreakable after-dinner evenings a week—replete with a favorite family dessert, suggest the experts. Can't spend the traditional Sunday in the park or backyard together because of other obligations? Then designate Friday evening as Family

Night—to rent a movie, visit a museum or help serve dinner at a homeless shelter. Not able to walk your son to school as your mother did with you? Then put daily notes—about what a great kid he is, the weather, a joke—in his backpack for him to read so he will feel connected with you.

For couples, consider weekends away ("rituals of renewal"), anniversary trips back to the place where you met and that old standby, weekly dinner dates. Or update this restaurant ritual by taking a Mexican cooking course. Buy season tickets to the local theater or ballpark. And don't overlook smaller, hokey-but-who-cares rituals that can have a big impact—giving each other flowers the first of the month, sending cards to each other's workplace and making a brief, daily "I love you" call. Revive the rituals you once shared as well—perhaps taking a bath together, dancing in the living room to old records, combing his hair, falling asleep curled together like two commas.

IT SOUNDS SO EASY, BUT . . .

Don't blame lack of time for not giving rituals your best shot, say family therapists. "Our ancestors didn't work any less hard than we," says William Taft Stuart, Ph.D., assistant chair of the Department of Anthropology at the University of Maryland in College Park, "but they took the time." After all, a tight schedule wouldn't explain why, during most weekends, members of modern families seem to have separate plans. If we really long for togetherness, couldn't we *make* time?

The answer may be that we are our own worst enemies. We've grown up in a go-go world that prizes change, speed, spontaneity. We know having rituals is good, but the word also brings notions about sameness, regularity—qualities we don't value.

We've gotten ourselves into a bad trap. What we've decided, whether we know it or not, is that the individual is more important than the couple or the family. We have our freedom, but the price is isolation; and the more distanced we are from one another, the more forced our rituals feel. The best rituals are really nothing more than a reflection of our desire to be close to one another. It's not rituals that are stiff; it's we who are awkward about all the cleaving together.

The key to overcoming this awkwardness is giving yourself over to simple rituals that are as idiosyncratic as you are. One father told me that he and his son have an acronym, HITYLTILY, short for "Have I told you lately that I love you?" The two use it with a hug or as a peace offering after a fight.

I've taken inspiration from my great-grandfather, who took an orange on a plate up to my great-grandmother every night of their life together. She brushed her hair while he peeled the orange with his silver penknife, always in one long, unbroken corkscrew curl of rind. Then they shared the orange and talked. Family lore has it that they never had a fight. I'm not sure I believe that, but I'm certain that they never went to bed angry.

—*Jennifer Allen*

MOMMIE DEAREST?

MOTHERS AND DAUGHTERS CAN BE THE BEST OF FRIENDS—OR THE WORST OF ENEMIES. THESE BASIC TECHNIQUES CAN HELP YOU REBUILD POSITIVE COMMUNICATION.

In the movie *Postcards from the Edge*, flamboyant ex-movie star Doris Mann, played by Shirley MacLaine, encourages her daughter, actor Suzanne Vale, to get up and sing before the crowd at a party Doris has thrown in her honor. Modestly and somewhat reluctantly, Suzanne, portrayed by Meryl Streep, obliges. Immediately afterward, Doris steals the show with a sassy number from her Vegas act—she even flashes her panties.

All her life, Suzanne has been upstaged by her mother. Doris also flirts with her daughter's dates and insists on answering for her when others ask questions. Finally, Suzanne blasts out at Doris: "Why do you always have to overshadow me?"

Competition between mothers and daughters (or between fathers and sons) is not uncommon, but sometimes it can indeed go over the top. It can start, say psychologists, when the daughter is a small child, an adolescent or an adult and can range in intensity from a mother's occasional put-down to a full-blown rivalry with the daughter over looks, career or other issues.

The competition often manifests itself in the mother's exaggerated need for attention, either from everyone in her vicinity—as is the case with Doris—or from her daughter specifically. A mother can also express competition through hostility and criticism or cool disinterest.

Competitiveness with peers is normal, notes Judith Coché, Ph.D., associate clinical professor of psychology at the University of Pennsylvania Medical School in Philadelphia. But trouble comes when a mother regards her daughter as a rival. "Not only is it inappropriate for a mother to judge her own worth or attractiveness by comparing herself with her adolescent or grown daughter," says Dr. Coché, "it's actually antithetical to what parenting is all about, which is nurturing—a giving of the self so that someone can go on to blossom in her own right."

A mother who was insufficiently nurtured herself, who feels insecure because as a youth she never received adequate love and attention, may feel competitive with and critical of her daughter, says Anne E. Bernstein, M.D., clinical professor of psychiatry at Columbia University College of Physicians and Surgeons in New York City. In addition, explains Dr. Bernstein, some mothers with low self-esteem may narcissistically consider their daughters extensions of themselves instead of independent individuals. This type of mother, says Dr. Bernstein, due to her own need for approval, tries to be perfect, and she regards her daughter as a showpiece. But if the "showpiece" daughter tries to *outshine* this mother, problems may arise.

It's important to realize that competitive mothers, in the

vast majority of cases, are not acting out of malice but rather are driven by their own insecurities and nonnurturing backgrounds. Be aware of how your mother was shaped by her upbringing and marriage, and how radically—in one generation—society's values have shifted regarding what a successful woman is. By gaining insight into your mother's behavior, you can boost your own self-esteem and help improve the all-important mother/daughter bond.

CRITICISM IN CHILDHOOD

Competition between mothers and daughters can begin when a daughter is very young, notes Natalie Schwartzberg, a family therapist on the faculty of the Family Institute of Westchester in Mount Vernon, New York. "In the marital relationship there's typically a negotiation over power [between the wife and husband]," she says, "and often [one of them forms] an alliance with one of the children. If an alliance is drawn between father and daughter—a 'father's little girl' situation—then what does the mother do? She's outside of a tight system. What people can do when pushed outside of a system is attack."

When a man shows more affection to his young child than to his wife, the wife may criticize the girl in hopes of undermining the father/daughter relationship or of getting back at the husband, says Dr. Bernstein.

"When I was a child, my mother wanted my father's full attention," says Laura, 27. "So behind his back, she put him down to me and my brothers to weaken our relationship with him, fundamentally so she could have him to herself."

Further proof that Laura's mother saw her daughter as a rival is the way she took over Laura's other relationships, never allowing the child her own moment in the spotlight. "When I was 7," Laura recalls, "I started playing the piano. I showed some talent, and I suspect my mother was jealous. She sat through every one of my lessons—*and* became best friends with my teacher, a woman. When we moved to another country and I studied with a man, she flirted with him outrageously. Suffice it to say that I quit when I was 12 because by that time I felt that music was *her* interest, not mine."

Laura understands the roots of her mother's neediness. "My mother had a tough childhood," she says. "She was an unplanned baby. Her father left the family when she was four, and her mother emotionally neglected her. Terrible patterns seem to get handed down in families."

Laura's mother couldn't get to the point where she could enjoy the fact that her daughter had satisfying activities and relationships—she had to take them away for herself, says Dr. Bernstein.

COMPETITION IN THE TEEN YEARS

As a daughter moves into her teen years, a mother with low self-esteem may look for affirmation of her attractiveness from inappropriate sources—such as her daughter's boyfriends.

A subtler and more common form of maternal competition occurs when a mother finds her teenage daughter's attractiveness and budding sexuality so threatening that she reacts by being overly restrictive, preventing the daughter from getting her first bra or wearing makeup because she doesn't want her to be a sexual person—and thus a competitor, says Dr. Bernstein.

"Women's chips in society continue to be youth and attraction," says Schwartzberg. "As long as a youthful appearance is what society values in a woman, it's natural for a mother to be [at least slightly] competitive with her daughter because the daughter is younger."

Carla, 34, remembers how her mother told her, at age 11, that she would not be allowed to shave her legs until she was 16. "By the time I hit junior high, this was really embarrassing. I have very dark hair. I looked like a gorilla. But my mother was firm. I was allowed to bleach my legs, not much of an improvement, but not shave. Thankfully my grandmother intervened and simply gave me an electric shaver."

By trying to keep Carla a child, her competitive mother was making sure her own sense of attractiveness would not be challenged. This is a function of the competitive dynamic, says Dr. Bernstein: A mother can't bear to let her daughter's attractiveness be acknowledged because she sees it as diminishing *hers*. The mother believes that if somebody else wins—succeeds or receives attention—she has to lose.

Other mothers who see their teenage daughters as rivals may denigrate their emerging sexuality. "I was a pudgy kid," says Janet, 34, "but in the eighth grade I turned pretty. My mother almost seemed to resent it. No matter how I dressed she always had some critical comment, like 'I don't care if you wear a brassiere or not—you don't have breasts anyway.' And once I started having boyfriends—and had only gone as far as kissing—she'd make comments suggesting I was promiscuous. I took it all to heart. To this day I'm very self-critical—about my looks, about my progress in my career, about everything."

WHO'S THE MOM?

Another form of competition that can surface in adolescence is when—in a role reversal—a mother abdicates her duties as mom and has her daughter take care of her and the rest of the family. The mother thereby unconsciously ensures that her daughter won't be a competitor.

When Karen, who is now 38, was only 14, her mother, Joan, newly divorced and working, made Karen the surrogate mom for the family—for her four younger siblings and, in many respects, for Joan herself. Karen was expected to baby-sit, bathe the children and put them to bed, plus do all the cooking and cleaning.

Karen didn't date during high school; however, her mother kept her apprised of her affair with a married man. "She'd show me the lingerie she'd bought to go away with him for the weekend, while I'd stay home and take care of the kids," says Karen. "Now that's a flip."

This type of role reversal is a fairly common pattern in single-parent families, observes Schwartzberg, particularly with eldest daughters. It can also occur in situations where the father is emotionally absent due to workaholism or other reasons, adds Dr. Bernstein. By making her adolescent daughter take on a maternal role, a competitive mother ensures that the teenager won't be a rival for male attention.

MOTHER VERSUS GROWN DAUGHTER

A mother's competitive behavior over male attention or nurturing can linger when her daughter reaches adulthood. But at this time a new area of competition emerges: a daughter's career.

"In our generation, we are not affirming our mothers' lives by following the marriage-and-family route in the same way they did," says Pat Karr-Segal, who is a psychiatric social worker at the Family and Children's Services in Ithaca, New York. Women's opportunities and expectations have changed dramatically in the last few decades, and many mothers who never worked out of the home have not welcomed society's new expectations of women. A mother who takes an interest in the way her adult daughter raises her kids and runs the house but then seems completely disinterested in her career may feel threatened, says Karr-Segal, by her daughter's pursuit of a life different from her own, and/or she may be envious of her daughter's work. By refusing to give her daughter credit for professional accomplishments, a competitive mother may be unconsciously trying to negate and sabotage those successes. Again, the daughter's success may make this mother feel inadequate.

"I know my mother would have been happier with me if I had gotten married and had babies, because then I would have been following in her footsteps," says Janet, who works as a playwright. "But instead I've chosen a life diametrically opposed to hers, and she treats it like a rejection. I wish she could take some credit for the success I am today."

Two years ago Janet's mother finally attended one of Janet's musicals. "When she got to the theater she was drunk," says Janet. "It was really out of character. From where I was sitting in the back of the house, I could see her passed out. She didn't see any of the show."

Recently Janet's mother shocked her by admitting that she had always wanted to be a writer herself. In Janet's mind, a lot of her mother's behavior began to fall into place. "Maybe she feels that since she didn't have a chance at writing, I shouldn't either."

According to Karr-Segal, even when mothers are supportive of daughters who have surpassed their own achievements, there's also often an undercurrent of "How dare you?" "Some mothers who feel they've had their own needs denied don't always give their daughters permission to find their own happiness," she says.

Many of these mothers were raised in a family and society that emphasized that their primary role in life was to be an obedient wife and raise a family, says Dr. Coché. The idea of fulfillment through a career may have been out of the question. Now they see their daughters earning money, professional satisfaction and prestige in a much wider world. "If the mother's greatest accomplishment was the frustration of standing behind a man," Dr. Coché continues, "it can be hard for her to handle her daughter's achievements."

THE COMPETITIVE-MOTHER LEGACY

Having a competitive mother can damage a woman's self-esteem and may interfere with her ability to establish other successful relationships. "A child's self-concept is [largely] a reflection of how her mother feels about her," explains Dr. Bernstein. "If a child and her mother have a good relationship early on, then when the daughter shifts her attention to her father, and then to boys and men, she will bring positive feelings to those relationships." However, if a daughter has a poor relationship with her mother, she often won't form a good relationship with her father or she will become so attached to him that it's hard for her to break away and become involved in mature love relationships. What's more, if a mother is insecure or bitter about men—factors that may help make her competitive with a daughter in the first place—her daughter may mirror these attitudes and approach men in an unsure or hostile fashion, says Dr. Coché.

Relationships with female friends and colleagues can also suffer when one has a competitive mom. "Once a daughter has broken loose from a difficult mother, she may not be willing to risk involvement and hurt with other women," says Dr. Bernstein. Another legacy of the competitive mom: the inability of a daughter to advance at work due to a poor self-image or because too much of her emotional energy is wrapped up in fighting old battles.

SETTING COMPETITION ASIDE

It's not unusual for a grown daughter to want to cut herself off from a competitive mother because she feels so angry and undermined. But this is usually not the solution, say the experts. "If you completely renounce a parent, it's like cutting off a part of yourself," says Karr-Segal. The goal, she points out, is to make the most of the connection you have.

"The remedy for being furious," adds Dr. Bernstein, "is to change the situation." Fury will fade once a supportive relationship has been established, she explains. If your mother is too emotionally troubled to meet you halfway, minimizing contact—not cutting it off—is often the wisest choice. Avoiding the problem usually makes the pain linger. Here are some techniques to help you ease your relationship with your mother.

Confront your feelings. "The important thing is to face your feelings, not deny them; to really confront the anger and hurt; and also be aware that this is *your* life now— not what your mother might want your life to be," says Schwartzberg. One step in this direction is to stop focusing on past grievances and concentrate on living in the present.

Understand your mother's history. You can defuse some of your anger, advises Schwartzberg, by looking objectively at your mother's behavior in the context of her family history and her marriage, including any traumas and sacrifices.

"Find out how the sons in her generation were treated as opposed to the daughters," says Karr-Segal. Was a college education for her encouraged? Did she, adapt well to society's changes brought on by the feminist movement? Or did she ignore them or feel that the rug was pulled out from under her? Has she had what you would consider a successful marriage?

Schwartzberg, who contends there is far too much "mother blaming" for disappointments in a daughter's life, tells women who are angry with their mother to be sure to examine the entire family situation, especially whatever role their father did or didn't play in their upbringing, and to recognize that most mothers who are now in their fifties or older had little power in the family and no encouragement to pursue a career. "The mother took care of most or all of the child-rearing," she notes. "The result is that she gets blamed for everything that went wrong in the family."

Avoid direct blame. When you have been angry and hurt for years by a competitive mom's behavior, it can be tempting to confront her with exactly how you feel. Accusations, however, rarely lead to favorable results. A broad statement like "You have ruined my life" may feel accurate to you, but it doesn't get you closer to your goal, which is communication and a peace pact. "It may be helpful for a daughter to talk about her childhood to her mother, but with objectivity and understanding about what caused the mother's behavior, never in a blaming way," says Schwartzberg. Once you accuse, she says, most people become defensive and shut down.

The idea, Karr-Segal adds, is not to express yourself to simply get things off your chest and score a victory but instead to present your case in a way that will enhance the relationship. When frictions arise, the most effective approach is to let your mother know that there is a problem in a gentle, clear manner. Express your hurt or frustration in "I" statements that don't put your mother on the defensive—such as "I feel so disappointed when my wishes about how we're going to spend the holidays aren't considered"—instead of an accusatory statement such as "You never consider my wishes when we make plans."

Monitor your own reactions. Watch how you react to your mother, starting with situations that are not so emotionally charged, such as a disagreement over where to go out to dinner, says Karr-Segal. "This way you can test out your own and your mother's ability to handle conflict. Do you feel you need to win or to put her down? Or do you find yourself feeling depressed or submitting very quickly? Though you can't change her behavior, you can change how you respond to it. Don't make the assumption that you have to react in the same ways as you have in the past." Also, when conflict arises, try to deal only with the issue at hand and not bring in old baggage, like "This is just like at Mary's wedding, when you insisted on complaining about how much you hated my hair."

Find common ground. Enjoy and emphasize whatever it is you share, Karr-Segal recommends—a taste in music, a similar stance on political issues, your ethnic heritage, an interest in decorating.

Assert yourself and set limits. When a competitive mother requires too much attention and tries to monopolize your time—repeatedly calling you at the office, for instance—it's important to establish guidelines. Let her know when she can call and how long you can speak, says Dr. Coché. "By setting limits and being honest about what is happening in the relationship at that given moment, a daughter won't end up feeling imposed upon and resentful."

Find other supportive relationships. If you do so, your relationship with your mother won't be so dominant, says Dr. Bernstein. In addition to turning to your husband or boyfriend or caring friends, be sure to reach out to relatives to enhance your sense of family.

Exercise and relax. To help diminish anger, says Dr. Bernstein, invest that energy into something worthwhile and productive—exercise, meditation and anything else that relieves tension.

WHEN ANGER PERSISTS

When self-help techniques such as those above don't help you resolve your anger, therapy may be needed to heal old feelings and hurts, says Karr-Segal. Therapy can help you to accept the fact that it's natural to feel disappointed and deprived because you never had a nurturing mother and recognize that you may have borne the brunt of the pain and unhappiness in your mother's life.

Therapy is also useful when a mother is so troubled and rigid that she is incapable of change. The therapist in these cases helps the daughter understand the family dynamics that shaped her mother and come to terms with the extent of her mother's limits.

"Realizing that she has a deeply troubled mother is, in my experience, one of the most difficult realities for a woman to accept," says Dr. Bernstein. "You have to recognize that this kind of mother has severe problems of self-esteem you can't fix. Trying to get her to give more is an impossible task."

Once a daughter reaches this awareness, Karr-Segal explains, she undergoes a grieving process, "mourning for the mother she had hoped for." However, the anger and sorrow eventually dissipate, says Dr. Coché. "The daughter becomes more forgiving of her mother's rigidities and realizes that her mother is doing the best she knows how; that if she knew how to do better, she would. The adult daughter becomes a kind of parent in the situation, taking her mother's emotional limitations into consideration rather than the other way around."

This is different from the unhealthy teenage role reversal mentioned earlier, because the daughter now has an adult's perspective.

At this point the adult daughter may also be able to see the gifts her mother did give her—whether "she taught you a love of books or gave you some very good genes in terms of appearance," says Dr. Coché.

"Some women will always feel they never got adequate nurturing, because in fact they never did," Dr. Coché continues. "Nothing can make up for that lack. However, therapy can go a long way toward establishing a life that feels full and satisfying. It can free up a daughter to get on with her life."

In spite of all the dissatisfaction that having a competitive mother can bring, a daughter's negative feelings are usually tempered by a deeper level of loyalty and love. "It's very hard for me to admit I'm angry with my mother, because I really do love her," says Janet. "Although we have difficulties, I realize that this world without her would be an extremely bleak and lonely place."

—*Michele Wolf*

ARE YOU A GOOD ROLE MODEL?

YOUR CHILDREN LOOK TO YOU FOR A VISION OF
THEIR OWN FUTURE. HERE'S HOW TO GIVE THEM
A POWERFUL AND POSITIVE MESSAGE.

Ann Turkel's daughter, Heidi, had a favorite game
when she was younger; she loved to "play psychiatrist."

"She'd sit in my chair and I'd be the patient," Turkel says.
"I'd tell her: 'I have this problem with my daughter. She
won't behave.' She'd say 'I don't like that problem. Give me
another one.' "

The game was not very surprising to Turkel, who is a
psychiatrist herself. She knew that Heidi was just trying to
see what it felt like to walk around in Mom's shoes.

Beth Rosen watches her daughter, Emily, and other first-
graders swing their knapsacks self-importantly on the way to
school. "They don't have anything they really need to carry.
But they all want a 'briefcase' like their parents have," says
Rosen, a psychotherapist in New York City. "Instead of playing house when they come home from school, they play
'work.' They tell their dolls, 'I have to go to work now. Try
to be good while I'm away. Bye-bye.' "

In a country full of working mothers, American children
are pioneering new ways to play grown-up, based on
women's changing roles. Experts say the experience of
watching Mommy go off to her job every day can have an
enormous impact on how kids view the world and their
place in it. Children draw conclusions about what it's like to
be a working mom, depending on the way they see their
mothers behave and talk about their jobs.

"Both boys and girls pay very close attention to how
their moms approach their career," says Kyle Pruett, M.D., a
clinical professor of psychiatry at the Yale Child Study
Center in New Haven, Connecticut. "They notice whether

you care about what goes on at work, and whether it gives you pleasure and joy."

Having a working mother who is a positive role model is particularly important to daughters. There's been increasing concern in recent years about the tendency of smart, confident, independent little girls to somehow lose their sense of self when they hit puberty.

"You see this very dramatic decline in some adolescent girls' perceptions of their competence," says Deborah Phillips, Ph.D., a psychologist at the University of Virginia in Charlottesville. Part of the problem seems to be that teenage girls find it hard to envision a positive future for themselves. They begin to notice that women's roles today are extremely complex and demanding—that they will be expected to do well both at home and in the workplace. They may feel overwhelmed, unless they see their own moms successfully handling these demands.

"There is evidence that when daughters see an example of a competent, self-supporting mother, they incorporate it into their view of what's possible for themselves," says Dr. Phillips. And other research reveals that the daughters of working mothers are more likely to pursue higher education and become high achievers in the workplace.

Seeing moms out in the work force—and dads sharing the household chores—also teaches kids they have many options in life. A child whose mother is both a policewoman and a bedtime-story reader and whose father is both an accountant and a grocery shopper is less likely to begin life burdened with sexual stereotypes. In one study, for example, children were given a list of jobs and activities, ranging from "be a doctor" to "climb a hill." Then they were asked "Who can do these things?" Kids with working moms were more likely than other children to give women credit for having diverse abilities—not just in employment, but also in hill-climbing and truck-driving, according to Lois Hoffman, Ph.D., a psychologist at the University of Michigan in Ann Arbor and a leading expert on the effects of maternal employment.

SHARE YOUR PLEASURES

What does all this mean to you? Put simply, you are your children's most important role model, so it's a good idea to closely examine what they are learning from you.

The crucial factor in becoming a positive role model, everyone agrees, is not how much you are achieving in the workplace but how you feel about being there. "The key here is whether the mother is happy with the choices she's made," says Marsha Weinraub, a psychologist and director of the Infant Behavior Laboratory at Temple University in Philadelphia.

A factory worker and a brain surgeon are on equal footing when it comes to this all-important variable. Kids don't have much sense of occupational status, but they sure understand whether Mom feels good about her life. And the more information you share with your children about the positive aspects of your job, the better.

"Work is about being useful to somebody. That's a concept children can easily grasp," says Dr. Pruett. "If you wash apples for a living, you can tell your youngsters: 'I go to the apple-packing plant. And I wash the apples so people don't get sick when they eat them. I really like watching the truck roll out, taking all the crates of apples to the store, and feeling I've been a part of it.' "

Talking enthusiastically about new tasks you plan to take on at work also sends a positive message. "You're showing them that what's over the next hill is inherently interesting and worth pursuing," says Dr. Pruett.

Many experts also say it's a good idea to take your children to your job to see where you work and what you do. "Do not assume for a minute that your kids don't care about where you go, who your friends are, what you have for lunch," says Dr. Pruett. Seeing what you do gives them a concrete vision of you in another role than Mommy, and ideas for their own future.

Kathy McCullough, a Northwest Airlines pilot from Wasco, Oregon, took her eight-year-old daughter, Darcie, to Japan on one flight. "Even if my daughter decided not to work outside the home," McCullough says, "at least she knows that she can do whatever she wants—that she has the option to be anything she wants to be."

McCullough also helps Darcie see a link between schoolwork and future careers. "When I help Darcie with her math homework, I explain how I need math in my job—to check the fuel gauges or mileage. I think it helps her understand that math does have concrete uses."

Children who accompany their parents to the workplace also gain a realistic view of what it takes to accomplish a goal. Susanne Bleiberg Seperson, a sociology professor at Dowling College in Oakdale, New York, has an office at home, which gives her children an intimate view of how she approaches her work. "They pick up on the fact that there's a lot of work to be done, that there are opportunities out there if you want to take them, that things don't happen by magic," Seperson says.

Independence is another lesson kids can learn from watching their mothers perform successfully in the workplace. "Children are infinitely impressed by behavior," says Dr. Pruett. "When a mom gets herself up, puts on her work clothes and goes out in the world to take care of people's needs, her kids receive a very strong message that it's good to be motivated and self-reliant."

Indeed, Elva Valentine, owner of a jewelry store in Dallas, Pennsylvania, says that when her son was 13 he became quite resourceful, even in the face of peer pressure. He admitted that his friends were making fun of him because he took the bus to the mall instead of having his mother drive him. "He said, 'They're the ones that should be made fun of—they can't get there by themselves,'" Valentine reports.

Pediatrician Chrystal de Freitas, of Ann Arbor, Michigan, also says her children have learned positive ways to be self-sufficient. On Mondays, Wednesdays and Fridays, her three children (ages nine, seven and six) come home to a caregiver and play together for a few hours. "Since my husband and I are not around 24 hours a day, the kids don't always look to us to settle conflicts. They negotiate among themselves and have learned to depend on and help one another," she says.

Being a working mother is, of course, not always fun or rewarding. And being a good role model does not mean covering up the difficult parts. "It's bad to give an unbalanced view," says Dr. Pruett. "It's not useful for kids to hear only the positive. There are some days when you don't want to get up—you're facing a hard meeting or a deadline. Kids can understand that."

WHEN WORK ISN'T REWARDING

Children also understand when you are truly unhappy with your job, whether you come right out and tell them or not. If you are often exhausted and stressed, or if you complain about the demands of your job, they are likely to feel less optimistic about their own future. They may conclude that work is a burden rather than an opportunity to be useful and self-supporting.

"One really interesting study involved girls who had fairly negative attitudes toward women's work. Their mothers were engaged in hard, unglamorous, unfulfilling jobs. And the daughters did not see working as the path to self-fulfillment," says Kristin Moore, director of Child Trends, a nonprofit research group in Washington, D.C. "Clearly, the message depends on whether the mother likes what she's doing."

That doesn't mean you have to pretend to love a job you loathe. Instead, show your children that it's possible to make positive changes when things are tough. If you feel you're underpaid, ask for a raise. If you need more time for your family, lobby for a flexible schedule. If things are truly miserable with your current employer, look for a new position.

But remember that your career is only one part of the picture. Children are also keenly aware of how life at home is going. "Sometimes what the children see is simply a very harassed woman," says Martha Haffey, clinical director of Co-Counsel, a therapeutic service for women. "She may be stressed because there isn't equal sharing of the homemaking tasks between husband and wife. But the kids don't know that's the problem." They may mistakenly conclude that it's bad for a woman to be employed outside the home.

When Marsha Weinraub and her colleagues at the Infant

Behavior Laboratory took a look at how two- and three-year-olds viewed gender roles, they found that the kids were heavily influenced by their fathers' actions. Children with dads who shared domestic chores were much less likely to cast men and women into old-fashioned roles and more likely to see it as perfectly normal for Dad to wash dishes and Mom to fix the car.

And the number of such children is growing as more and more mothers take on jobs outside the home. Pilot Kathy McCullough, for example, says that her husband takes over the household and child-care chores when she's away on flights. "It's good for the kids to see dad vacuuming, doing the laundry, giving baths and changing diapers. I think my son—who often imitates my husband's vacuuming—will grow up understanding that it's not right for the woman to do most of the work at home. And I think my daughter will know to marry someone who is willing to help with housework and child care. She'll know that it's hard for one person to do everything," says McCullough.

Her experience is far from unique. When mothers and fathers feel good about their lives, children see their parents as positive role models. "The most wonderful statistic I ever found in maternal-employment literature is that daughters of working mothers are more likely than other girls to name their mother as the woman they most admire," says Weinraub.

That's exactly what happened to Charlotte Kielminski, a manager for Cooper Lighting in Elk Grove Village, Illinois. Her daughter, Kelly, was asked if she'd like to be a fashion model when she grows up. "Kelly said, 'No. I want to do what my mom does. She has a great job, and I'd like to work at Cooper Lighting when I'm older.' Her answer really surprised me," says Kielminski. "But it sure made me feel good!"

Susanne Bleiberg Seperson recounts a similar story: During a parents' night program in her daughter's sixth-grade classroom, the teacher asked the kids to tell who their heroes were. "When my daughter picked me," Seperson says, "I was stunned. She said, 'Mom, I know how hard you work. I know what you do for us. I want to be like you.' I was melting."

—*Gail Collins*

CREDITS

PART ONE

"**A New Era for Women's Health**" by Leslie Laurence was originally published in *Glamour*, June 1992. Copyright © 1992 by Leslie Laurence. Reprinted by permission.

"**Six Diseases Doctors Miss**" by Susan Chollar was originally published in *McCall's*, April 1993. Reprinted with permission of *McCall's* magazine. Copyright © 1993 by the New York Times Company.

"**Take the Ache Out of Backache**" by Sheila Sobell was originally published in *Woman's Day*, May 1992. Copyright © 1992 by Sheila Sobell. Reprinted by permission.

"**The Headache Handbook**" by Saralie Faivelson was reprinted from *Ladies' Home Journal*, March 1992. Copyright © 1992 by Meredith Corporation. All rights reserved. Reprinted by permission.

"**Staying Well in a Sick Building**" first appeared in *Working Woman*, January 1993. Written by Linda J. Murray. Reprinted with permission of *Working Woman* magazine. Copyright © 1993 by Working Woman, Inc.

"**A New View of Your Menstrual Cycle**" by Lisa Couturier was originally published in *New Woman*, February 1993. Copyright © 1993 by Lisa Courturier. Reprinted by permission.

"**In Search of a Good Night's Sleep**" by Dava Sobel was originally published in *Allure*, February 1993. Copyright © 1993 by Dava Sobel. Reprinted by permission.

"**The Ten Most Important Health Questions You Can Ask**" by Leslie Laurence was originally published in *Glamour*, April 1993. Copyright © 1993 by Leslie Laurence. Reprinted by permission.

PART TWO

"**Why It's So Tough to Lose Those Last Ten Pounds**" was reprinted from *The Last Ten Pounds* by Linda Konner. Copyright © 1991 by

Linda Konner. Reprinted by permission of Longmeadow Press, Stamford, Connecticut, and Linda Konner.

"Six Simple Rules for Eating Right" by Daryn Elder was originally published in *McCall's*, June 1992. Reprinted with permission of *McCall's* magazine. Copyright © 1992 by the New York Times Company.

"Can the Fat Imposters Fake Out Your Taste Buds?" first appeared in *Working Woman*, June 1992. Written by Robert Barnett. Reprinted with permission of *Working Woman* magazine. Copyright © 1993 by Working Woman, Inc.

"Diary of a Demanding Diner" by Susan V. Seligson was reprinted from *Health*, October 1992. Copyright © 1992 by *Health* magazine. Reprinted by permission.

"Shortcuts to Fitness" by Michael Castleman was originally published in *First for Women*, April 1993. Copyright © 1993 by Michael Castleman. Reprinted by permission.

"I'd Kill for a Cookie" by Beth Weinhouse was originally published in *Redbook*, August 1992. Copyright © 1992 by Beth Weinhouse. Reprinted by permission.

PART THREE

"Stress Busters That Work" by Laura Flynn McCarthy was originally published in *Woman's Day*, April 1992. Copyright © 1992 by Laura Flynn McCarthy. Reprinted by permission.

"How to Get Rid of That Tired Feeling" by Richard Laliberte was originally published in *McCall's*, April 1993. Reprinted with permission of *McCall's* magazine. Copyright © 1993 by the New York Times Company.

PART FOUR

"Forever Younger Skin" by Shirley Lord was originally published in *Vogue*, August 1992. Courtesy *Vogue*. Copyright © 1992 by The Condé Nast Publications, Inc.

PART FIVE

PART SIX

PART SEVEN

PART EIGHT

"**Exercise for Fun (for a Change)**" by Mary Talbot was originally published in *Allure*, November 1992. Copyright © 1992 by Mary Talbot. Reprinted by permission.

"**How to Beat the Time Crunch**" by Kelly Good McGee was originally published in *New Woman*, January 1993. Copyright © 1993 by Kelly Good McGee. Reprinted by permission.

PART NINE

"**What Men Can't Get from Women**" by Tom Lowry was reprinted from *Ladies' Home Journal*, January 1992. Copyright © 1992 by Meredith Corporation. All rights reserved. Reprinted by permission.

"**Private Wars of Loving Couples**" by Sonya Rhodes was originally published in *McCall's*, April 1993. Reprinted with permission of *McCall's* magazine. Copyright © 1993 by the New York Times Company.

"**Is Your Husband Sexually Insecure?**" by Kate Nolan was originally published in *Redbook*, July 1992. Copyright © 1992 by Kate Nolan. Reprinted by permission.

"**Frank Answers to 22 Sex Questions**" by Avodah K. Offit, M.D., was originally published in *Mademoiselle*, July 1992. Copyright © 1992 by Avodah K. Offitt, M.D. Dr. Offitt is the author of the book *The Sexual Self.*

PART TEN

"**The Incredible Healing Power of Family Rituals**" by Jennifer Allen was originally published in *McCall's*, February 1993. Reprinted with permission of *McCall's* magazine. Copyright © 1993 by the New York Times Company.

"**Mommie Dearest?**" by Michele Wolf was originally published in *New Woman*, December 1992. Copyright © 1992 by Michele Wolf. Reprinted by permission.

"**Are You a Good Role Model?**" by Gail Collins was originally published in *Working Mother*, April 1993. Copyright © 1993 by Gail Collins. Reprinted by permission.

INDEX

Bait-and-switch scams, 166–67
Behavior
    changes, 186–87
        maintenance, 194–95
        stages of, 90–94
    competition in marriage, 244–48
    sexual roles, 240
    at work, 127–30
Benzoyl peroxide, for skin care, 120
Beta blockers, for migraines, 25
Bicycling, as exercise workout, 227
Bills, debt reduction and, 177–85
Biofeedback
    for back pain, 20
    for headache, 26
Birth control pills, 8
Bisexuality, 260, 261
Blackheads, 120
Blood pressure, high. *See* High blood pressure
Body image, 205–6
    advertising and, 251–52
Body size, weight loss and, 63
Bone health, 50–51
Boxing, as exercise workout, 223–25
Brain, intuition and, 210–11
Breast cancer
    detection, 3, 13
    family history and, 46, 47
    genetic research on, 9–10
    soy and, 6
Budget
    debt reduction and, 180
    planning, 157–58

Buildings, air quality in, 29–32
Business. *See* Career; Work
Butter, in restaurant meals, 76, 77

C

CA 125 blood test, for ovarian cancer, 3
Caffeine, sleep and, 109
Calcium
    in diet, 66–67
    for osteoporosis prevention, 50
    premenstrual syndrome and, 7
Calcium channel blockers
    for cluster headaches, 27
    for migraines, 25
Calories, low-fat foods and, 69–70
Cancer. *See also specific types*
    chemotherapy for, 9
    detection, 2–3
    family history and, 46
    from smoking, 53
Carbohydrates
    cravings for, 90, 93
    for sleep, 108
Career. *See also* Work
    advancement, 143–49
    competition between spouses, 244–48
    of daughters, 274–75
    goals, 132–40
    reduced sexual interest and, 253
    role models and, 281, 282–85
Cars. *See* Automobiles
Changing behavior. *See* Behavior, changes

THE HEALTHY WOMAN

Depression
    negativism vs., 197
    severe, 204–5
    symptoms, 11
DHE, for migraines, 22,
    25
Diabetes, conception and,
    51
Diagnosis of disease
    disagreeing with, 12
    inaccurate, 10–14
Diet. *See also* Dining out
    healthy changes in,
        47–48
    high-carbohydrate, low-
        fat, 7
    principles, 65–67
Dieting. *See also* Food crav-
    ings; Overweight; Weight
    loss
    losing last ten pounds,
        60–65
    yo-yo, 5, 61–62, 93
Dihydroergotamine (DHE),
    for migraines, 22, 25
Dining out, healthy, 71–81
    tips for, 78–79
Disability insurance, 159
Discounts, advertised, cau-
    tions about, 166–67
Disease, missed diagnoses of,
    10–14
Down's syndrome, alpha-
    fetoprotein test for, 52
Dreams (lifestyle), fulfilling,
    132–40

E

Economics. *See* Finances
Ejaculation, premature, 259
Elavil, for migraines, 25

Emotions
    anger toward mother,
        276, 277, 278–79
    awareness of, 190
    backache and, 18–20
    change and, 189
    premenstrual syndrome
        and, 37, 38
Endometrial cancer, 8
Endometriosis, RU 486 for, 8
Endorphins, food cravings
    and, 92, 93
Erection difficulty, 249, 253
Ergotamine, for migraines,
    25
Estrogen, osteoporosis and,
    6
Ethnic foods, healthy dining
    and, 80–81
Etidronate, for osteoporosis,
    9
Exercise. *See also* Walking
    aqua-aerobics, 226–27
    boxing, 223–25
    cycling, 227
    duration and intensity, 5
    excuses for avoiding,
        83–84
    for fun, 222–29
    funk and hip-hop,
        225–26
    gym classes, 223
    for heart health, 4–5
    for insomnia, 44–45
    low-intensity, 82–83
    program, 49–50
    sleep and, 106–7
    yoga, 228–29
Extrasensory perception,
    210–11
Eye creams, excessive use of,
    118

F

Facial masks, 119
Facial skin, 112–17, 117–21
Family
    change and, 189
    rituals, 264–69
Family history, health and,
    46–47
Fantasies, sexual, 257, 259
Fashion trends, 121–23
Fat (body), weight loss and,
    62–63
Fat (dietary)
    cravings, 89, 93
    reducing, 66, 69, 70–71
    in specific foods, **69**
    substitutes and low-fat
        foods, 67–71
    weight loss and, 5–6
Fatigue, sleep and, 103–6
Feminism, men's movement
    and, 241, 242, 243
Fertility, 48–49
Finances
    auto repairs, 168–77
    budget, 157–58
    debt reduction, 177–85
    goals and, 157
    insurance, 158–59
    investment plan, 159–60
    professional opinions
        on, when to seek, 156,
        157
    retirement savings, 160
    savings plan, 158, 159
    scams, 163–68
    scrimping, 160–63
    self-management of,
        155–60
Fires, in home, 55
Fitness shortcuts, 82–88

Folate, in pregnancy, 52
Food cravings, 88–95
    healthy ways to handle,
        90–91
Food, meditation on, 6
Foreplay, 256
Funeral costs, cautions
  about, 165

G

Gay relationships
    female, 261
    male, 260
Genealogy book scams, 165
Genetic disorders, 51–52
Genetic tests, 47
German measles, pregnancy
  and, 51
Glycolic acid peels, for skin
  care, 114–15
Goals. *See also* Behavior,
  changes
    financial, 156
    lifestyle, 132–40
    self-esteem and, 203
Gym classes, 223

H

Headaches
    causes of, 23–24
    cluster, 27–28
    costs of, 22–23
    migraine (*see* Migraines)
    posttraumatic, 28
    secondary, 24
    sinus, 28
    tension-type, 26–27
    TMJ, 28
Health
    disease diagnosis, 10–14

Health (*continued*)
    questions, 45–57
    screening tests, 13
    self-esteem and, <u>203</u>
Health care for women, federal funding of, 56–57
Health insurance, 159
Heart disease
    exercise and, 4–5
    missed diagnosis of, 13
    prevention, 46
    weight cycling and, 61
Herbs, for insomnia, 42–43
High blood pressure
    in pregnancy, 7–8, 51
    reduced by modest exercise, 82–83
Home, time management at, 232–33
Homeowners' insurance, 158–59
Home scams
    mortgage payments, 164
    real estate, 166
    repairs, 168
    working at home, 167–68
Homosexuality
    female, 261
    male, 260
Hormones, menstruation and, 37, 38
Household chores, husband sharing, 285
Hydroquinone, for skin care, 115
Hypertension. *See* High blood pressure

I

Ibuprofen, for backache, 16
Imagery
    intuition and, 214
    for success, <u>202</u>
Impotence, male, 249
Income. *See also* Salary
    debt and, 179
Independence, children learning, 283
Indian food, healthy dining and, 80–81
Insomnia, 40–45, 104. *See also* Sleep
    acupuncture and herbs for, 42–43
    from alcohol, 42
    exercise for, 44–45
    sleep labs and, 41
    sleep restriction for, 44
Insulin resistance, diet and, 7
Insurance, types of, 158–59
Intercourse, 256–57, 258. *See also* Sex
Interest rates, debt reduction and, 182, 184
Interferon, for skin cancer, 55
Interruptions, time management and, 232
Interviews, job, 147
Intrauterine devices, 48
Intuition, 209–15
Investments, 159–60
Iron, for sleep, 108
Iron deficiency, food cravings and, 92, 93

J

Jewelry, buying, 167
Jobs. *See* Career; Work

K

Karate, as exercise workout,
224–25

L

Lesbian relationships, 261
Life insurance, 158
Lifestyle
    calling/dreams, 132–40
    changing, 188–96
    of mother vs. grown
        daughter, 274–75
Lithium, for cluster
    headaches, 27
Loan scams, 164
Lung cancer, 53–54
Lyme disease, 10–11

M

Malignant melanoma, 4, 54
Mammograms, 3, 47
Marriage
    competition in, 244–48
    sexually insecure hus-
        band, 248–55
Masculinity
    new view of, 240–41
    sexual insecurity and,
        249
Mastectomy, phantom pain
    and, 9

Materialism, self-esteem and,
    202
Meat cravings, 92
Mechanics, automobile,
    168–77
Meditation
    on food, 6
    for self-esteem, 203
Meetings, time management
    and, 233
Melanin, for skin care, 112
Melanoma, 4, 54
Men's movement, 238–43
Menstruation, 32–40. *See also*
    Premenstrual syndrome
    attitudes toward, 33–36,
        39
    cycle, stages of, 37–38
    easing pain of, 36
    lifestyle and, 39–40
    sex and, 38–39
Metabolism, weight loss and,
    63
Methysergide, for migraines,
    25
Midrin, for migraines, 29
Migraines, 21–22
    diagnosis, 11–12
    symptoms, 24–25
    treatment, 25–26
Milia, eye creams and, 118
Modeling, child, 167
Moisturizing, excessive,
    117–18
Money. *See* Finances
Mortgage payments
    debt reduction and, 178,
        180, 182, 184
    foreclosure threats, 164

Mothers. *See also* Role models
  fitness tips for, 88
  relationship with daugh-
    ters, 269–79
Motor vehicle accidents,
  55
Moving cost estimates, cau-
  tions about, 165
Muscle injuries, 56
Music, for stress, 101
Mutual funds, 159

N

Nail biting, 188
Negative thinking, 196–99,
  203. *See also* Self-esteem
    self-assessment test, 198
Neural tube defects, folate
  and, 52
Noise, sleep and, 106, 107
Nutrition principles, 65–67

O

Obesity. *See* Overweight
Obstetrics, 52–53
Oral contraceptives, 8
Oral sex, 257, 258
Orgasm, 252–53, 256
  faking, 257
Osteoporosis
  estrogen and, 6
  etidronate for, 9
  prevention, 50–51
Ovarian cancer
  detection, 2–3
  family history and, 46
  new treatment for, 9
Overeating, at restaurants,
  78–79

Overweight. *See also* Dieting;
  Weight loss
    food cravings and,
      93–94
    genetic predisposition
      for, 63
Oxygen therapy, for cluster
  headaches, 27

P

Parenting, stress from, 102–3
Pay increases, obtaining,
  140–43
Peer pressure, in children, 283
Personal appearance, 112–23
  mother-daughter com-
    petition and, 272–73
Pessimism, 196–99, 203. *See
  also* Self-esteem
    self-assessment test, 198
Petroleum jelly, for skin care,
  116
Pets, for stress, 101
Phantom limb syndrome, 9
Phone calling cards, cautions
  about, 165
Phone conversations, time
  management and, 233
Phytoestrogens, breast can-
  cer and, 6
Pica, during pregnancy, 93
Pimples, 120
Positive thinking, 203. *See
  also* Negative thinking
Preeclampsia, 7–8
Pregnancy, 7–9
  food cravings, 92–93
  prenatal care, 51–53
Premature delivery, 7–8
Premature ejaculation, 259

Premenstrual syndrome,
34–35, 36
  calcium and, 7
  emotions and, 37, 38
  food cravings and, 91–92
  sleep and, 105
Prenatal care, 51–53
Privacy deprivation, 218–22
Products and services
  complaint letters about,
    152–55
  ripoff protection, 163–68
  store return policies, 164
Protein, 66
Prozac
  for depression, 205
  for migraines, 27, 29

Q

Quiétude, for insomnia, 43

R

Radio frequency trigeminal
  gangliorhizolysis, for cluster headaches, 27–28
Raises (pay), obtaining,
  140–43
Real estate agents, cautions
  about, 166
Rectal examination, digital, 3
Relationships. See also Family;
  Spouses
  change and, 189
  competition in
    husband-wife,
      244–48
    mother-daughter,
      269–79
  homosexual, 260, 261

Relaxation. See also Stress
  intuition and, 214–15
Reproductive health, 7–9
Resolutions, how to keep,
  188–96
Restaurants, healthy dining
  in, 71–81
Retin-A, for skin care, 113,
  114–15
Retirement savings plan,
  160
Ripoff protection, 163–68
Rituals, family, 264–69
Role models, 280–85
Rollerblading, as exercise
  workout, 227–28
RU 486, for endometriosis, 8

S

Salary
  getting better-paying
    job, 143–49
  obtaining raises, 140–43
Salt
  basic desire for, 89
  cravings, 90–91, 94
  in diet, 67
Sansert
  for cluster headaches, 27
  for migraines, 25
Scams, protection from,
  163–68
Screening (health) tests, 13
Self-discovery, 132–40. See
  also Behavior, changes
Self-esteem, 200–208
  body image and, 205–6
  boosting, 202–3, 206–8
  in children, 281, 283
  defining, 200–201

Self-esteem (*continued*)
  lack of, 201, 204
  mother-daughter com-
    petition and, 270–72,
    275–76
Serotonin
  food cravings and,
    91–92, 93
  headaches and, 23
Sex
  answers to questions
    about, 255–61
  insecure husband and,
    248–55
  menstruation and, 38–39
  orgasm (*see* Orgasm)
  roles, 240, 251
Sexually transmitted disease,
  8–9, 260
  condoms and, 48
  pregnancy and, 51
Sexual stereotypes, 281,
  285
Shoes, for exercise, <u>86</u>
Sick building syndrome,
  29–32
Sickle-cell anemia, prenatal
  test for, 51
Silva Method, for relaxation,
  214–15
Sinus headaches, 28
Skin, younger, 112–17
Skin cancer, 54–55
Skin-care mistakes, 117–21
Sleep, 103–9
  problems, 107 (*see also*
    Insomnia)
  quality, 104–6
  stages, 105
  strategies for better,
    106–9

Smoking, 53–54
  vitamin C and, 7
Sneakers, choosing, <u>86</u>
Soap, skin and, 118
Solicitors, uninvited, cautions about, 164–65
Solitude, lack of, 218–22
Soy
  breast cancer and, 6
  in Chinese restaurants,
    81
Spine-care centers, 17
Sports injuries, 56
Spouses
  competition between,
    244–48
  rituals for, 266, 268
  sexually insecure hus-
    band, 248–55
Steaming, for skin care,
  119
Stimulants, sleep and, 109
Stock investments, 159,
  166
Stomach upset, sleep and,
  108
Stress
  cravings and, <u>91</u>
  evening, 100–101
  food and, 94
  illness and, 220
  intuition and, 214–15
  midday, 99–100
  morning, 98–99
  parental, 102–3
  from privacy depriva-
    tion, 220–21
  reducing, 98–103
  sexually insecure hus-
    band and, 248–55
  walking for, 83, 99

THE HEALTHY WOMAN